An Atlas of
INFECTIVE ENDOCARDITIS

THE ENCYCLOPEDIA OF VISUAL MEDICINE SERIES

An Atlas of
INFECTIVE
ENDOCARDITIS
Diagnosis and Management

C. Ward

North West Regional Cardiothoracic Centre
Department of Cardiology
Wythenshawe Hospital
University of Manchester School of Medicine
Manchester, UK

With contributions from

P. Hasleton
B. Isalska
N. Stanbridge

Wythenshawe Hospital
University of Manchester School of Medicine
Manchester, UK

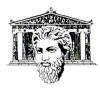

The Parthenon Publishing Group
International Publishers in Medicine, Science & Technology

NEW YORK   LONDON

British Library Cataloguing in Publication Data
Ward, C.
  Atlas of Infective Endocarditis:
  Diagnosis and Management. —
  (Encyclopedia of Visual Medicine Series)
  I. Title II. Series
  616.125

  ISBN 1-85070-462-7

Library of Congress Cataloging-in-Publication Data
Ward, C.
An atlas of infective endocarditis: diagnosis and management
/ C. Ward
    p.   cm. — (The Encyclopedia of visual medicine series)
Includes bibliographical references and index.
ISBN 1-85070-462-7
I. Infective endocarditis—Atlases. I. Title. II. Series.
[DNLM: I. Endocarditis, Bacterial—diagnosis—atlases.
  WG 17 W257a 1995]
RC685.E5W37 1995
616.1'1—dc20
DNLM/DLC
for Library of Congress   95-745
                                                    CIP

Published in the UK and Europe by
The Parthenon Publishing Group Limited
Casterton Hall, Carnforth
Lancs, LA6 2LA

Published in the USA by
The Parthenon Publishing Group Inc.
One Blue Hill Plaza,
PO Box 1564, Pearl River,
New York 10965, USA

Copyright © 1996 Parthenon Publishing Group Ltd

First published 1996

Typeset by Keele University Press, Staffordshire, UK
Printed and bound by TG Hostench S.A., Spain

Contents

Foreword   7

Acknowledgments   9

Section 1   A Review of Infective Endocarditis   11

Section 2   Infective Endocarditis Illustrated   35

Section 3   Bibliography   89

Index   93

The Encyclopedia of Visual Medicine Series

Titles in this series include:

An Atlas of Oncology

An Atlas of Hypertension

An Atlas of Common Diseases

An Atlas of Osteoporosis

An Atlas of the Menopause

An Atlas of Contraception

An Atlas of Endometriosis

An Atlas of Ultrasonography in Obstetrics and Gynecology

An Atlas of Practical Radiology

An Atlas of Psoriasis

An Atlas of Trauma Management

An Atlas of Lung Infections

An Atlas of Transvaginal Color Doppler

An Atlas of Infective Endocarditis

An Atlas of Rheumatology

An Atlas of Epilepsy

An Atlas of Differential Diagnosis in HIV Disease

An Atlas of Practical Dermatology

An Atlas of Laser Operative Laparoscopy and Hysteroscopy

An Atlas of Atherosclerosis

An Atlas of Eye Diseases

An Atlas of Cutaneous Growths

An Atlas of Myocardial Infarction

An Atlas of Diabetes Mellitus

Foreword

Infective endocarditis has always attracted much more attention from students of medicine than its incidence in the population would suggest. One reason is its ability (as with tuberculosis and syphilis) to involve virtually any organ and masquerade as many different diseases. Another is the fact that it is uniformly fatal without treatment but is usually curable with therapy.

The disease has changed dramatically over the past 50 years. Among these alterations are changes in organisms, predisposing disease, clinical manifestations, diagnostic tools, therapy and outcome. There is much less pneumococcal and gonococcal endocarditis, much more staphylococcal disease and a recognition of *Streptococcus bovis* infection with its association with gastrointestinal malignant and premalignant disease. Rheumatic heart disease has become much less common as an underlying disease and has been replaced by prosthetic valves, mitral valve prolapse (previously unrecognized), and intravenous drug abuse as predisposing conditions. Lack of significant murmurs has become more common due to the increased incidence of intravenous drug abuse (where tricuspid valve involvement is common) and prosthetic valves as underlying conditions. Tricuspid valve endocarditis and prosthetic valve endocarditis may present without murmurs. Many other clinical manifestations such as splenomegaly, petechiae, Osler nodes, and clubbing have become much less frequent probably due to earlier diagnosis and therapy.

Improved blood culture techniques have resulted in higher yields, and the advent of echocardiography, especially transesophageal echocardiography, has enhanced diagnostic capabilities.

Development of newer antimicrobial agents along with cardiac surgical techniques has resulted in cure of many cases which previously would have been fatal. More recently, home therapy has become widespread using agents such as once a day ceftriaxone or twice a day vancomycin.

An Atlas of Infective Endocarditis reviews the clinical spectrum of infective endocarditis and covers many of the current aspects. The greatest strength of the Atlas is the 92 figures, many in color, which demonstrate the pathology, clinical manifestations and diagnostic techniques in endocarditis.

Donald Kaye, MD
Klinghoffer Professor of Medicine, Department of Medicine, Medical College of Pennsylvania & Hahnemann University,
and
President and CEO
Medical College of Pennsylvania & Hahnemann University Hospital System,
Philadelphia, Pennsylvania, USA

Acknowledgments

We would like to thank our colleagues who have kindly lent slides for this atlas:

Drs Margaret Aird (Figure 26), David Beton (Figures 43, 50–53, 69), Colin Bray (Figures 31–38), Robert Henderson (Figures 77–79) and Andrew Horrocks (Figures 9, 11, 22–24, 92).

Also the following pharmaceutical companies who have given permission for publication of slides from educational material:
    Boehringer Ingelheim (Figures 42–49)
    Zeneca Ltd. (Figures 7, 8)
    Leo Laboratories (Figure 17)

Finally we wish to thank members of the Department of Medical Illustration, Wythenshawe Hospital, Manchester, UK, who produced most of the figures used and Mrs C. Darnley who typed and prepared the manuscript.

Section 1   A Review of Infective Endocarditis

Introduction   13

Historical notes   15
  A changing disease   16

Pathogenesis   17

Diagnosis   19

Symptoms and clinical findings   21
  Effects of infection and septicemia   21
  Cardiac involvement   21
  Emboli   23
  Central nervous system involvement   23
  Renal involvement   24
  Cutaneous and other peripheral
    manifestations   24
  Differential diagnosis   24

Investigation   25
  Microbiological investigation   25
  Echocardiography   27
  Other investigations   28
  Immunological responses and effects   28

Problem cases   29
  Prosthetic valve endocarditis   29
    Clinical features   29
  Fungal endocarditis   30
  Intravenous drug users   31
  Chronic renal failure   31
  Infective endocarditis in the elderly   31
  Culture-negative endocarditis   32
  Conclusion   32

Clinical management   33
  Late deaths   34

Introduction

Infective endocarditis has fascinated and challenged doctors for more than 200 years. This is not surprising as it is a condition which may, on the one hand, present with a long history of vague ill health or, on the other, with acute severe cardiac failure. It has bizarre and diverse clinical manifestations and is invariably fatal without the correct treatment. It is, however, not a common condition. A generous estimate of the incidence of infective endocarditis in the United Kingdom would be 3000–4000 cases a year. In the North West Regional Cardiothoracic Centre at Wythenshawe Hospital, we see 20–30 cases per year. The average general practitioner may see only one or two cases in a working lifetime. It is this infrequency, combined with the varied and vague presentation of infective endocarditis, which provides the challenge. The mortality has remained stubbornly at between 20% and 30% for several decades, although we have available diagnostic techniques, antibiotics and surgical skills which together could reduce the mortality to less than 10%. But reduction in mortality will only be achieved by earlier diagnosis and the prompt institution of appropriate treatment. It is a sobering fact that approximately one in five cases are not diagnosed during life.

Another intriguing aspect of infective endocarditis is the way in which the disease appears to have evolved as our attempts to treat it have improved. For example, having found effective antibiotics to treat the viridans group of streptococci, we are now seeing an increasing number of cases caused by staphylococci, a worrying number of strains of which are resistant to the penicillins; and the introduction of valve replacement surgery has provided us with the new challenge of prosthetic valve endocarditis.

Writing shortly after the early successes of treating infective endocarditis with penicillin, Dr Paul White, a pioneering American cardiologist, observed, 'Thus we continue to grope for a specific cure, having made a slight but definite step forwards in the past few years.' Since then, we have made several additional steps forward but have perhaps also accepted that vigilance will do more to improve the prognosis than searching for a specific cure.

Historical notes

An Italian physician, Lazarus Riverius, is credited with the earliest description of infective endocarditis. In 1646, he described the postmortem findings in a man who had died from cardiac failure. 'In the left ventricle … round carbuncles were found … which resembled a cluster of hazelnuts and filled up the opening of the aorta.' Although other graphic descriptions followed, Bouillard in 1841 was the first to recognize the condition as a form of endocarditis and clearly to distinguish it from rheumatic endocarditis. Shortly after this, Virchow in 1847 observed that the vegetations were not, as was generally stated, simply depositions of fibrin. In one autopsy study, he described vegetations on the posterior mitral valve cusp. 'On this a ragged, fringed, hanging, fibrous coagulum 4 inches long … in some places degenerated into a reddish, pus-like pulp.' The next major advance was made by a Norwegian pathologist, E. F. H. Winge, in 1869. He gave the first indication that infective endocarditis was of bacterial origin when he saw under the microscope 'short rod-shaped or round bodies' in what he described as 'a parasitic vegetation'.

In 1885, Sir William Osler lectured on the subject of malignant endocarditis. This, and his subsequent writings, provide a marvellous overview of the pathogenesis and clinical features of infective endocarditis. Most of his observations are still valid today.

Epidemiological studies in the opening decades of this century showed clearly the toll which infective endocarditis took on the lives of patients with rheumatic and congenital heart disease; it was responsible for up to one-third of all deaths in these groups. A fatal outcome was virtually inevitable and resulted from sepsis, emboli and cardiac failure with anemia an important contributing factor. Dr Paul White found that, of 250 well-documented cases, only one survived, although other workers reported cures by ligation of an infected patent ductus arteriosus, and a few others were attributed to the use of antimeningococcal and antipneumococcal sera. The therapeutic use of sulfonamides was very disappointing but the introduction of penicillin in the early 1940s was dramatically effective. Cure rates of 75–85% were claimed – better than in some recent reports! This is at least partly because they took no account of relapses, recurrences and subsequent deaths from cardiac failure. Nevertheless, this was a turning point in the treatment of infective endocarditis, and, in terms of lives saved and prolonged, it outweighs any subsequent innovation.

Since that time, progress has been in four main areas:

(1) More diverse antibiotic therapy. The most commonly used antibiotics in the treatment of endocarditis are penicillin or ampicillin for streptococcal infections and flucloxacillin for β-lactamase-producing staphylococci. Vancomycin is used as an alternative to the β-lactam antibiotics in penicillin-allergic patients.

In the treatment of Gram-negative infections that are ampicillin-resistant, the cephalosporins have proved valuable, especially the third generation cephalosporin, ceftazidime, which has activity against *Pseudomonas* spp.

Aminoglycosides may be used for their synergistic activity with the penicillins in the treatment of staphylococcal and streptococcal infections, or for their Gram-negative activity.

Fungal infections remain a problem. Intravenous amphotericin B is moderately effective, but surgical removal of the valve is usually needed to obtain a cure. Recently introduced amphotericin formulations and the newer imidazole antifungals may improve the effectiveness of medical treatment.

In addition, microbiological techniques have improved. Assays of antibiotic levels and assessment of minimum inhibitory/bacteriocidal concentrations have placed antibiotic treatment on an objective basis.

(2) A better understanding of the pathogenesis of the disease.

(3) Improved diagnostic techniques, notably echocardiography.

(4) Valve replacement surgery. The first valve replacement operations for cardiac failure caused by infective endocarditis were in the early 1960s. The operative mortality for this previously fatal complication is now only 10–25%.

A changing disease

It would not be unreasonable to assume that, as a result of the advances mentioned – more antibiotics, better diagnostic facilities and open heart surgery – the mortality from infective endocarditis would have continued to fall. This has not happened: the overall mortality is still approximately 25%, similar to the figure about 40 years ago. However, if we look at the typical patient being treated for infective endocarditis in the 1930s and 1940s (young, female, with mild

mitral regurgitation and infected with a viridans streptococcus), the mortality for such patients today is only 5%; on the other hand, if we look at a cross-section of today's patients, we see a different picture. The average age has increased and aortic valve endocarditis is much more common, as is staphylococcal infection. Each of these factors is independently associated with a poor prognosis and is partly responsible for the continuing high mortality. There are also specific problems associated with endocarditis in immunocompromised patients and drug addicts. In addition, we have 'invented' a new disease, namely prosthetic valve endocarditis. This accounts for 15–20% of cases and has a mortality in the region of 50%.

Pathogenesis

Endocardium consists of endothelium and the underlying connective tissue. Normal endothelium is highly resistant to bacterial invasion, and is present as a continuous layer of flattened cells. With laminar blood flow, the nuclei of these cells are arranged in parallel lines. This alignment is lost when blood flow changes direction or when there is turbulence. This altered pattern may be seen, for example, along the lines of valve closure and some of these areas may become denuded of endothelial cells. Non-bacterial thrombotic vegetations, consisting of platelets and fibrin, form at these sites of endothelial trauma, and have been described in 1–2% of routine postmortem examinations. Non-bacterial thrombotic vegetations occurred especially in patients with congenital and acquired cardiac defects and also in patients who have malignant disease, disseminated intravascular coagulation, or who are on dialysis. Infective endocarditis is initiated when bacteria adhere to these vegetations. Several factors have been identified which it is thought may promote bacterial adhesion to non-bacterial thrombotic vegetations. These include:

(1) The production of dextran by viridans streptococci (non-dextran-producing strains adhere poorly to a platelet–fibrin matrix in experimental animals);

(2) Fibronectin which binds to collagen exposed by endothelial injury and for which receptors are present on, for example, *Staphylococcus aureus* and several types of streptococci;

(3) The ability of staphylococci and streptococci to aggregate platelets; and

(4) Activation of clotting mechanisms by some organisms.

Thus, there are three phases to the development of infective endocarditis – endocardial damage, adherence of microorganisms to the damaged endocardium, and multiplication of the implanted organisms.

The hemodynamic factors related to the development of infective endocarditis are:

(1) A high-velocity jet stream,

(2) Flow from a high- to a low-pressure chamber, and

(3) A narrow orifice between chambers.

These factors may explain the predilection for vegetations to form at certain sites; in patent ductus arteriosus it is usually on the pulmonary artery, at the point where the jet of blood from the ductus impinges, in mitral regurgitation on the atrial aspect of the mitral valve and in aortic regurgitation on the ventricular aspect of the aortic valve. At each of these sites the Venturi effect ordains maximum turbulence and so a likelihood of microtrauma. The frequency with which the different valves are affected (mitral valve most often, then aortic, tricuspid and pulmonary), correlates with the relative mechanical stress to which each valve is subjected.

Diagnosis

Infective endocarditis is not a common condition. What makes it important is that delayed treatment results in irreparable damage, and, if untreated, it is fatal. Approximately 3 000–4 000 cases occur each year in the United Kingdom. This means that the average family doctor will see a case only once every 8–10 years. Add to this the vagueness of the symptoms (*see* below) and we have a simple explanation for the fact that, for several decades, the time from the onset of symptoms to diagnosis has remained at approximately 10 weeks. The vagueness and non-specific nature of the symptoms also explain the even more worrying fact that, in up to 20% of cases, the diagnosis is not made during life. The difficulty in diagnosing infective endocarditis was emphasized in 1885 by Sir William Osler: 'It is important to recognize the manifold conditions under which the disease may present'. He also wrote about 'the different modes of onset and the extraordinary diversity of symptoms which may arise … the general symptoms are those of a febrile affection …' and 'in a considerable number of cases, the heart symptoms remain in the background, hidden by the general condition'. It is fascinating to note that, 99 years later, in the same Journal (*The Lancet*), an editorial begins with the words 'Infective endocarditis is hard to diagnose, hard to treat and hard to prevent.' For all of these reasons, a high degree of suspicion is essential if the diagnosis is to be made promptly – bearing in mind

that the longer the delay in instituting treatment, the more extensive is valve damage. The diagnosis of infective endocarditis, like that of many conditions, passes through three stages:

(1) Suspicion,

(2) Supportive clinical findings, and

(3) Confirmation.

Part of the process of suspecting infective endocarditis requires an awareness that some groups of patients are at an increased risk of developing the disease because of pre-existing conditions. The list includes patients with malignant disease, diabetes, collagen vascular disease, chronic renal failure, and those having steroid therapy or hyperalimentation. In immuno-suppressed patients and drug addicts, previously normal valves may be affected. Others are at risk because they have a focus of infection, for example, dental caries, those who have had recent surgery, osteomyelitis, skin infections, sinusitis, intravenous lines, arteriovenous shunts, and pneumonia. Enquiries should always be made for a possible iatrogenic cause for the infection. For example, bacteremia occurs during urethral surgery and periodontal operations in 50–70% of cases and in 30–45% of tooth extractions and tonsillectomies. However, while 50% of patients with enterococcal endocarditis may report prior genitourinary manipulations, no source of bacteremia is found in 85% of cases of non-enterococcal streptococcal endocarditis.

Symptoms usually begin within 2 weeks of an initiating bacteremia.

A high level of suspicion can be maintained if the diagnosis is always considered in certain clinical settings:

(1) Pyrexia in a patient with a heart murmur or prosthetic heart valve;

(2) Vague ill health in a patient with a murmur or prosthetic valve (in fact, unexplained vague ill health even in the absence of heart murmurs);

(3) Unexplained worsening of cardiac failure, recurrent pulmonary emboli or pneumonia, systemic emboli or normochromic anemia; and

(4) Any patient with a positive blood culture.

Of course, in many instances, there may be an obvious alternative explanation for patients in each of these categories. But an awareness of the possibility of infective endocarditis in these situations should then prompt a search for the often subtle supportive clinical findings. Unfortunately, some recent reports suggest that the incidence of the classical clinical findings is much less than is stated in standard accounts of infective endocarditis (Table 1).

Table 1 Incidence of clinical findings: pre- and post-1960s

	Pre-1960s	Post-1960s
Murmurs	95–99	85
Pyrexia	95	75
Splenomegaly	80–90	30
Petechiae	80	20–40
Finger clubbing	25–30	10–20
Osler nodes	70	10–15
Splinter hemorrhages	50	15–20

Symptoms and clinical findings

The manifestations, symptoms and clinical findings associated with infectious endocarditis result from:

(1) The direct effect of infection/septicemia,

(2) Valvular or cardiac damage,

(3) Emboli, and

(4) Immunological phenomena.

The classification of infective endocarditis into acute and subacute cases is based on observations made in the pre-antibiotic era. 'Acute' referred to cases which were fatal within a few weeks. Often the infected valve had been previously normal and the responsible organisms were virulent pathogens, e.g. *Staphylococcus aureus*, *Streptococcus pneumoniae* or *Haemophilus influenzae*. Infected emboli were common. On the other hand, subacute endocarditis involves previously abnormal (usually rheumatic) valves infected with commensal organisms such as the viridans streptococci. In these cases the patient sometimes survived for more than a year. Nowadays, most cases no longer fit neatly into these subgroups, and so the classification has been largely abandoned.

Effects of infection and septicemia

The infection gives rise to pyrexia in more than 90% of cases, although some recent reports suggest an increase in the number of apyrexial cases – 25% in one series. Possible explanations for this include the prior use of antibiotics and the observation that the 'normal' temperature in the elderly is relatively low and may thus be elevated but still within the 'normal' range. Patients with cardiac or renal failure are also sometimes apyrexial, probably for the same reason.

Rigors occur in approximately 50% of cases and are more common when the onset is acute.

Other features which accompany chronic sepsis may be present and include anorexia, weight loss (perhaps largely due to muscle wasting), pallor, anemia, and splenomegaly. Septicemia frequently causes tachypnea, myalgia, arthralgia and occasionally arthritis – the latter usually with sterile synovial fluid. Adult respiratory distress syndrome can occur and may be incorrectly diagnosed as pulmonary edema.

Cardiac involvement

The incidence of rheumatic heart disease began to decrease in the United Kingdom during the latter part of the nineteenth century and the rate of this decline accelerated in the first three decades of this century. Consequently, rheumatic heart disease as a substrate for infective endocarditis has declined. Nowadays, mitral valve prolapse, degenerative aortic and mitral valve disease and congenital heart disease are more common. In fact, more patients have no detectable underlying heart disease than have rheumatic heart disease. Congenital heart disease is responsible for 10–20% of cases, the commonest forms being patent ductus arteriosus, ventricular septal defect and a bicuspid aortic valve. The predisposing lesions in infective endocarditis are shown in Table 1.

Table 1 Lesions predisposing to infective endocarditis

Lesion	Responsible for infective endocarditits (%)
Mitral valve prolapse	20–50
No known heart disease	25–50
Rheumatic heart disease	20–30
Degenerative valve disease	30 (age > 65 years)
Congenital heart disease	10–20

Data from Braunwald, E. (1992). *Heart Disease. A Textbook of Cardiovascular Medicine*, 4th edn. (Philadelphia, London, Toronto, Montreal, Sydney, Tokyo: W.B. Saunders)

At one time, a diagnosis of infective endocarditis would not have been considered if there was no heart murmur but now, depending to some extent on the population being studied, between 10 and 15% of cases may not have a murmur during the early stage of the infection – these are usually acute cases and/or patients with tricuspid valve endocarditis. A murmur, of course, does not necessarily indicate advanced valvular damage. It is, at least in the early stages, merely a marker of a susceptible lesion. Although changing murmurs are supposed to be characteristic of infective endocarditis, this is neither a common nor a sensitive diagnostic criterion, a changing murmur is more likely to be due to alterations in the heart rate or in cardiac output in a patient who is pyrexial for some other reason, rather than because of progressive valve damage caused by infective endocarditis.

It is a fallacy to equate the intensity and duration of murmurs with the severity of valve damage. This is particularly relevant to acute valve lesions such as rupture of an aortic or mitral valve cusp or of the chordae tendineae. In the case of acute severe aortic regurgitation, the classical clinical signs of a collapsing pulse and a long blowing early diastolic murmur are often replaced by a low blood pressure, a weak pulse and a short, early diastolic murmur – the latter because the left ventricular end-diastolic pressure rises dramatically, causing the aortic and left ventricular end-diastolic pressures to equate early in diastole, thus terminating the murmur. Similarly, the murmur of severe acute mitral regurgitation may be limited to early systole because of the dramatic increase in left atrial systolic pressure with the onset of ventricular contraction. However, in both situations, there will be clinical and radiological evidence of cardiac failure and echocardiography will demonstrate severe valvular regurgitation.

It cannot be overemphasized that, in the vast majority of cases, the onset or progression of cardiac failure provides the best and often only clinical indication of the extent of damage caused by the infection. With very few exceptions, cardiac failure results from the destruction of valvular tissue or perforation of a valve cusp – in mitral valve endocarditis ruptured chordae tendineae may be the cause. Detection of early signs of cardiac failure requires daily clinical assessment, regular chest X-rays and, when indicated, repeated echocardiography (see below). As a general rule, cardiac failure is an indication for urgent valve replacement; if this fact was more widely recognized and acted upon, then the mortality in infective endocarditis would be much less. Cardiac failure is responsible for almost two-thirds of all deaths.

Other less common cardiac complications include:

(1) *Coronary embolus*: this may contribute to cardiac failure or give rise to the typical clinical pictures of myocardial infarction.

(2) *Myocarditis and myocardial abscess*: both are still quoted as contributing to cardiac failure but are rare causes. Myocardial abscesses are detected at

postmortem examination in approximately 20% of cases, but are usually very small and are of doubtful significance. In practical terms, cardiac failure should never be attributed to myocarditis since this may lead to neglect of a surgically remediable valve lesion.

(3) *Periannular abscess*: this occurs in up to 25% of cases of native valve endocarditis, notably when infection involves the aortic valve, and this may be accompanied by a pericardial rub and by electro-cardiographic evidence of atrioventricular block. A periannular abscess is always present in prosthetic valve endocarditis. In both native and prosthetic valve endocarditis, it is a cause of persistent pyrexia despite apparent appropriate dosages of suitable antibiotics. Detection is by echocardiography and is often an indication for early surgery.

(4) *Purulent pericarditis* is fortunately rare. The patient remains severely toxic despite appropriate antibiotics. Echocardiography indicates pericardial effusion but it should be noted that a small effusion is not uncommon in infective endocarditis. Pericardio-centesis is needed to confirm the purulent nature of the fluid. Open (surgical) drainage is usually necessary.

(5) *Rupture of sinus of Valsalva*: this is an uncommon but well-recognized complication. The right coronary sinus and the non-coronary sinus are involved in a ratio of 2 : 1; it is exceptionally rare for the left coronary sinus to be involved. Rupture occurs usually into the right atrium or the right ventricle. This is accompanied by a continuous murmur, best heard at the left sternal edge and is associated with the development of cardiac failure. Echocardiography will detect the site of the lesion and also indicate the chamber into which rupture has occurred. Surgical correction is required. Although rupture of a sinus of Valsalva is a dramatic event, it does not always lead to a sudden deterioration in the patient's condition – in almost 50% of cases, progressive cardiac failure occurs only gradually.

Emboli

Clinical evidence of emboli is present in 20–30% of patients and in up to 60% of cases in postmortem studies. Major emboli are most likely when the infection is caused by organisms which produce large friable vegetations – for example, fungi and *Staphylococcus aureus*. Whether the embolus produces infarction or an abscess depends on whether or not the embolic material is infected. Emboli from left-sided lesions are randomly distributed throughout the circulation. Emboli from right-sided endocarditis produce pulmonary infarctions, abscesses or pneumonia. As noted above, emboli are often clinically silent. When symptoms occur, they produce the expected clinical picture of embolization to that site, occurring in other conditions, for example, splenic infarction, bowel ischemia from mesenteric embolism or peripheral arterial occlusion. Major emboli, usually cerebral, are responsible for 20% of deaths.

Central nervous system involvement

This requires specific mention for several reasons:

(1) Extensive cerebral damage is often permanent and is an important cause of death;

(2) Emergency treatment may be required to treat or to prevent a ruptured mycotic aneurysm or a space-occupying lesion such as a cerebral abscess; and

(3) The presence of an intracerebral hemorrhage precludes open-heart surgery because of the need for anticoagulation during the operation.

Up to 20% of patients present with evidence of central nervous system involvement. This will obviously cause diagnostic difficulties when it is recalled that increasing numbers of patients present without a heart murmur. Most neurological features are embolic and usually involve the territory of the middle cerebral arteries. The majority of the remainder have vertebrobasilar insufficiency. Emboli are often multiple and so patients with cerebral emboli often have others elsewhere.

Mycotic aneurysms may be single or multiple – it is important to appreciate this when contemplating surgical treatment. Quite often, rupture of a mycotic aneurysm is heralded by severe focal headache. Other prodromata include meningoencephalitis and transient ischemic attacks.

Symptoms of an acute toxic encephalopathy is the second most common neurological feature of infective endocarditis and patients occasionally present in this way. It may manifest as drowsiness, confusion, irritability or apathy. This is especially common in the elderly. The pathology is multiple microinfarctions secondary to emboli. Macroabscesses (>1 cm) are not common, nor is meningitis. Other uncommon neurological features include back pain and mononeuropathies.

Subarachnoid and intracerebral hemorrhage are uncommon presenting features.

Renal involvement

Renal emboli are common. They may be small and multiple, causing microscopic hematuria and 'flea-bitten kidney' or large, causing severe loin pain and marked hematuria.

Focal glomerulonephritis is a rather common but trivial complication of infective endocarditis. Diffuse proliferative glomerulonephritis is less common but much more serious. Current thinking is that they represent two extremes of the same disease process. Both are common in untreated cases, the diffuse and focal form in 33% and 50%, respectively. However, both are rare in fatal cases if given penicillin.

Diffuse proliferative glomerulonephritis has an overall incidence of 10% in fatal cases and is often associated with a positive rheumatoid factor (see below), cryoglobulins and reduced levels of C3 – suggesting an immune-mediated disease. Immunohistology shows deposition of IgG, C1q, C3 and C4 in the glomerular basement membrane – typical of circulating immune complex injury. This is seen usually with prolonged infection, especially due to streptococci.

Cutaneous and other peripheral manifestations

These are important, not because of their frequency (which has declined in recent years) but as an aid to diagnosis. However, none of these 'classical' signs is pathognomonic with the possible exception of Roth spots.

Petechiae are common, occurring in 20–40% of cases. They are found not only on the limbs but also on mucous membranes. Other lesions, splinter hemorrhages, Osler nodes, Roth spots, Janeway lesions and subconjunctival hemorrhages are much less common.

Splinter hemorrhages, linear dark red streaks beneath the nails, occur in 20% of cases. Osler nodes are painful, red nodules usually in the finger pads and occur in 15% of cases. They persist for a few hours to a few days. Janeway lesions are less common. They are flat, hemorrhagic and non-tender lesions usually 1–4 mm in size on the palms of the hands or soles of the feet. Roth spots are oval retinal hemorrhages with pale centers. They are only found in 5% of cases.

There are several reasons for the decline in incidence of these features. First, they are typically found in subacute cases, whereas more and more patients now are presenting acutely. Second, the course of the disease is now modified by antibiotics and by surgery. The incidence of finger clubbing has declined for the same reasons.

Differential diagnosis

Because of the diversity of presentations of infective endocarditis, a complete list of differential diagnoses is a pointless exercise. However, a handful of conditions can give rise to a syndrome clinically indistinguishable from infective endocarditis; these include, atrial myxoma, non-bacterial thrombotic endocarditis, acute rheumatic fever, systemic lupus erythematosus, thrombotic thrombocytopenic purpura and sickle cell disease.

Investigation

Laboratory confirmation of the diagnosis of infective endocarditis relies mainly on microbiology and echocardiography. The role of microbiology does not only consist of the isolation or identification of the responsible organism, but also an assessment of antibiotic susceptibility. A further important aspect is the assay of blood antibiotic levels to ensure adequate therapeutic levels and to minimize the likelihood of toxic side-effects. However, laboratory testing in infective endocarditis is not simply to confirm the diagnosis. It is essential to the ongoing assessment of the patient to:

(1) Indicate if valve damage and/or cardiac failure is progressive;

(2) Indicate which valve(s) are affected;

(3) Help in the timing of valve surgery;

(4) Assess the nature and extent of damage caused by emboli; and

(5) Monitor renal damage.

Microbiological investigation
In infective endocarditis, organisms are shed constantly into the blood from the bacterial vegetation, and thus blood culture is central to the diagnosis and the subsequent antibiotic management of the patient. The bacteremia is independent of pyrexia and therefore blood cultures may usefully be collected on three separate occasions over the course of several hours. There is little to be gained from taking further blood cultures because, if an organism is to be recovered, in 90% of cases the isolate will be obtained from the first two blood samples.

Many publications have drawn attention to the importance of the volume of blood collected and the conditions of incubation. Laboratories vary in their blood culture protocols but most recommend the collection of 10–20 ml-aliquots at each venepuncture and its distribution into aerobic and anaerobic culture media. When collecting blood for culture, venepuncture must be performed with strict attention to asepsis in order to minimize casual contamination. Laboratories may also use special techniques in order to obtain isolates, such as the use of diphasic media, pour plates and resin or enzyme-containing media to inhibit antibiotic present in the patient's blood.

There are a variety of techniques for the detection of bacteria or fungi in the blood culture and modern automated systems are based upon the recognition of changes in impedance, redox potential and the detection of carbon dioxide, either as the radioisotope (Bactec) or by infrared spectrophotometry (Bactec) or by colorimetric methods (Bact/Alert).

Broths should be examined within 24 h and then again at intervals for up to 3 weeks before being discarded after a final subculture. Those suspected of being positive are examined by Gram's stain and sub-cultured onto appropriate media which are incubated in CO_2-enriched and anaerobic atmospheres. Special cultural conditions are required for the isolation of some fastidious organisms such as nutritionally-deficient strep-tococci and *Legionella*. Organisms are isolated in approximately 90% of patients with endocarditis. Culture-negative patients should be screened by serology for *Coxiella* (Q fever), *Chlamydia*, *Brucella* and *Legionella*.

Positive blood cultures must be interpreted in the context of the clinical setting, as contamination of the culture by skin flora may easily occur unless strict attention is paid to aseptic technique during the collection of the blood sample. The antibiotic sensitivity of isolates must be fully determined by means of the minimum inhibitory concentration, minimum bactericidal activity and *in vitro* assessments of the likely synergistic or antagonistic effects of combinations of antibiotics.

Although almost all species of bacteria have been implicated as etiological agents of endocarditis, the vast majority of native valve infections are due to oral and gut streptococci and to *Staphylococcus aureus*. The bacteria causing prosthetic valve endocarditis are more diverse but infections occurring within 12 months of surgery are usually initiated at the time of the operation and are caused by staphylococci (both coagulase-positive and coagulase-negative), *Candida* and diphtheroids, whereas, in late prosthetic valve endocarditis, the organisms are similar to those causing native valve endocarditis. Endocarditis following the insertion of pacemakers or intravenous catheters is nearly always due to staphylococci, and endocarditis in intravenous drug abusers is mostly due to *S. aureus* or *Pseudomonas* spp.

Streptococci can now be classified by their cultural, biochemical, cell-wall or DNA characteristics. These developments have led to a revision of their nomenclature, and recently to the assignment of enterococci (formerly *Streptococcus faecalis* or *faecium*) to the genus enterococcus. It is therefore possible to consider the streptococci causing infective endocarditis as belonging to one of four broad groups – the oral strep-tococci or viridans group, the enterococci, the pyogenic group and the pneumococcus.

The oral streptococci remain the commonest causative organisms of native valve endocarditis, responsible for up to 40% of culture-positive cases. They consist of a number of different species, many of which produce α-hemolysis when grown on blood agar, but some produce either no hemolytic effect or, rarely, a β-hemolysis of the medium. The three most common organisms in this group are:

(1) *S. sanguis*: its ability to produce dextran from sucrose enables it to adhere to the platelet–fibrin meshwork as the vegetations are being formed;

(2) *S. mutans*: interest in this organism was reawakened when it was shown to produce dextran and to be involved in the production of dental caries; and

(3) *S. oralis* (*S. mitior*): also a mouth organism of which approximately 25% of isolates produce dextran.

The enterococci form part of the normal bowel flora and are responsible for up to 20% of cases of endocarditis. The incidence is increasing, perhaps because of the increased use of invasive investigation of gastrointestinal pathology in an aging, susceptible population.

S. bovis deserves special mention. It is responsible for 15–20% of cases caused by streptococci and is a commensal organism of the gastrointestinal and genitourinary tracts. It has some characteristics of the enterococci (e.g. group D antigen) but, unlike them, it is very sensitive to penicillin. An association between endocarditis caused by *S. bovis* biotype I and underlying bowel pathology, in the form of a malignant or premalignant lesion, has been shown in up to 75% of patients with endocarditis caused by this organism. These patients should therefore be investigated to confirm or exclude bowel pathology.

The pyogenic streptococci, which includes those possessing the Lancefield group antigens of A, B, C or G, and the pneumococci are rarer causes of infective endocarditis. They usually cause an illness with an acute, as opposed to a subacute, clinical course.

Echocardiography

Vegetations appear as echogenic masses attached to a valve. The early form of echocardiography (M mode) provides a one-dimensional display of cardiac function and demonstrates vegetations of 3 x 2 mm or greater in approximately 55% of cases. Structural abnormalities are better seen with two-dimensional (2D) echocardiography. Not only will this technique show similar-sized vegetations in 70–80% of cases, but it will also indicate their location, shape, and mobility (it is important to remember that the apparent size of vegetations depends to some extent on their echogenicity, the more reflective vegetations looking larger). The addition of continuous and pulsed-wave Doppler techniques to 2D-echocardiography provides yet more information, since with it an estimation of valve stenosis, based on flow rate, and valvular regurgitation can be made. A further refinement has been made by the addition of color coding to the Doppler signals, which provides valuable information about the direction of blood flow in a semiquantitative form as well as indicating when there is turbulence. Despite these improvements, both M mode and conventional (transthoracic) 2D-echocardiography are seriously limited in the information they provide, especially with respect to small vegetations, paravalvular abscesses, mycotic aneurysms and prosthetic valve endocarditis.

Transesophageal echocardiography overcomes many of these problems. With this technique, because the transducer is closer to the heart, the sound waves are less attenuated. Also, the employment of a transesophageal probe permits the use of a higher-frequency beam and thus high-resolution images are obtained. As a result, transesophageal echocardiography detects vegetations in approximately 95% of cases of native valve endocarditis. Prosthetic valves are highly echogenic and this may obscure echoes from other structures. However, for the reasons given, transesophageal echocardiography detects vegetations in at least 75% of cases of prosthetic valve endocarditis, compared with only 25% for transthoracic echocardiography and thus this technique should be used in all cases of suspected prosthetic valve endocarditis.

There are a number of intracardiac infective complications of infective endocarditis. The commonest of these is a paravalvular abscess which appears, echocardiographically, as an echo-free space, adjacent to the base of the valve. Other intracardiac complications are paravalvular mycotic aneurysms, cusp perforation, chordal rupture and valve dehiscence. Transesophageal echocardiography may demonstrate these pathologies in up to 80% of cases.

It is important to appreciate that the presence of vegetations does not imply that they are 'active', since, in up to two-thirds of cases, they remain unchanged despite successful treatment. Consequently, serial echocardiograms are required in order to document the size and shape of vegetations in the chronic healed stage.

There are a number of intracardiac pathologies which may, from time to time, be confused with vegetations. Such diagnostic pitfalls include thickened calcified valves or nodules, tumors, ruptured chordae, flail cusps and thrombus. These present less of a problem with transesophageal echocardiography.

Two specific clinical situations in which echocardiography is particularly useful are:

(1) Bacteremia without clinical signs of infective endocarditis – this accounted for almost 20% of cases in one series; and

(2) Culture-negative endocarditis.

The use of echocardiography in infective endocarditis may be summarized as:

(1) The detection and localization of vegetations;

(2) The assessment of extent of valvular damage;

(3) The assessment of perivalvular damage; and

(4) The detection of abscess formation, valve dehiscence, cusp rupture, and chordal rupture.

It should be stressed that, despite the sensitivity of transesophageal echocardiography, the inability to demonstrate vegetations echocardiographically does not exclude the diagnosis of infective endocarditis. If the diagnosis is thought likely despite a negative echocardiogram, treatment should be instituted and the test repeated after some days.

Other investigations

At one time, angiography was performed on most patients with infective endocarditis – it was used to demonstrate which valves were damaged, the extent of the damage and the state of the left ventricle. Perivalvular abscesses could sometimes be identified, as could aortic aneurysms. This information can now be obtained non-invasively with echocardiography. Consequently, left ventriculography is now only required if clinical examination and echocardiography give inconclusive evidence regarding the severity of lesions, which is very unusual. Furthermore, many cardiologists wish to avoid passing a catheter through an infected aortic valve because of the risk of detaching a part of the vegetation. However, coronary angiography may be required if there is concern about the presence of coronary artery disease.

A normochromic anemia is common and parallels the duration of the illness. The white blood count is often normal, although with a shift to the left. Leukocytosis occurs in the more acute cases. The erythrocyte sedimentation rate is raised. The level of C-reactive protein is a simple, rapidly performed assay which accurately reflects improvement or deterioration in a wide range of pathologies. In infective endocarditis, falling levels indicate control of infection, and rising levels, failure to do so. The levels of C-reactive protein change more quickly in response to changes in the clinical condition of the patient than do levels of immune complexes (see below) or the erythrocyte sedimentation rate. Evidence of renal damage is very common, but is only occasionally of clinical significance. Urinalysis often shows proteinuria, hematuria and/ or pyuria. The possible causes are cardiac failure, emboli/infarction or immune complex nephritis (see page 24). The importance of regularly checking the

blood urea in connection with antibiotic treatment is noted on page 33.

Serial chest X-rays form an important part of the assessment of any patient with infective endocarditis, first for the detection of evidence of pulmonary congestion, and second, in the case of right-sided endocarditis, for evidence of pulmonary infarction, pneumonia or abscess formation.

Computerized tomography (CT) has revolutionized the investigation of intracranial pathology. With respect to the complications of infective endocarditis, CT readily distinguishes between hemorrhage, infarction and abscess formation because these lesions cause different degrees of attenuation of the X-ray beam. Hemorrhage produces high attenuation and a white image, while infarction causes low attenuation and a dark or black image. An abscess typically shows a dark area surrounded by a white ring.

Abdominal ultrasound or CT can be used to detect or confirm intra-abdominal emboli. CT, but not ultrasound, will distinguish abscess formation from embolic infarction.

Immunological responses and effects

Prolonged bacteremia stimulates the immune system. A cellular response is indicated by circulating macrophages and by splenomegaly. The humoral response gives rise to a wide range of antibodies and also to a non-specific hypergammaglobulinemia. Circulating immune complexes are found in 95% of patients, high titers correlating with the duration of illness and a fall in titers with appropriate treatment. Titers are higher in these patients than in others with septicemia but without infective endocarditis. Persistently high levels, or a secondary rise, equate with continuing infection. Most patients with prosthetic valve endocarditis also have high titers of circulating immune complexes.

Fifty per cent of patients have a positive rheumatoid factor which is probably an 'anti-antibody' directed against the IgG of the circulating immune complexes, the levels of which increase before the rheumatoid factor does.

Problem cases

There are a number of situations in which infective endocarditis presents particular difficulties, either because of the nature of the infection or because of specific problems relating to a group of patients. Included under the heading are prosthetic valve endocarditis, fungal endocarditis, chronic renal failure, culture-negative endocarditis, the elderly, and intravenous drug users.

Prosthetic valve endocarditis

Prosthetic valve endocarditis is responsible for approximately 15% of all cases of infective endocarditis. It is a serious disease with a mortality of 50–80% and with differences from native valve endocarditis which make diagnosis more difficult. Patients with prosthetic valves are more at risk of developing infective endocarditis than are patients with damaged native valves. Depending on diagnostic criteria and the patient groups studied, the incidence is 0.5–0.9% per patient per year. The reasons for this high incidence are that non-bacterial thrombotic vegetations are inevitable around the sutures of the artificial valve and that abnormal flow patterns are produced by the prosthetic valve. These conditions encourage bacterial colonization (see section on pathogenesis, p18). Colonization always begins in the sewing ring around the valve, although with bioprostheses, the cusps may be involved. Calcification of a bioprosthesis increases the risks of non-bacterial thrombotic vegetations.

Prosthetic valve endocarditis is, by tradition, divided into 'early' (within 60 days of operation) and 'late' (> 60 days postoperation), although some consider all cases occurring within the first postoperative year as 'early'. Just as the microbiology of native valve endocarditis has changed over the years, so has that of prosthetic valve endocarditis. The changes are probably related to altered antibiotic prophylaxis, different perioperative care and a change in the patient population. Early prosthetic valve endocarditis is caused by organisms which gain entry at the time of surgery or in the perioperative period – for example, from intravenous lines or urinary catheters. In late prosthetic valve endocarditis the pattern of infection is similar to that found in native valve endocarditis.

Clinical features

Although the clinical features of prosthetic valve endocarditis and native valve endocarditis are broadly similar, there are important differences:

(1) Septic emboli are more common in prosthetic valve endocarditis, occurring in a third of cases in some series. This has been attributed to the turbulence associated with the prosthesis which is said to encourage the growth of large vegetations;

(2) Leukocytosis is more common;

(3) Anemia is less common; and

(4) Since patients with prosthetic valves often have left ventricular impairment – because of their history of pre-existing heart disease, often with episodes of cardiac failure – they develop cardiac failure more quickly with the hemodynamic burden imposed by the endocarditis.

Diagnosis is based on the presence of septicemia plus evidence of involvement of the valve ring or bioprosthetic valve. Infection progresses along the suture line (see above) and leads to a paraprosthetic leak. Thus, the development of a regurgitant murmur is highly significant, although in a small percentage of cases there may be evidence of valvular stenosis caused by a build-up of vegetation and thrombus causing obstruction to the valve orifice.

Transesophageal echocardiography can be regarded nowadays as almost mandatory in a patient with suspected prosthetic valve endocarditis (transthoracic echocardiography demonstrates vegetations in only 25% of cases but transesophageal echocardiography will demonstrate vegetations in 75–100% of cases – with a claimed predictive accuracy of 95%).

The diagnosis of early prosthetic valve endocarditis is particularly difficult because of the general clinical setting of a patient recovering from major surgery. In such patients, the differential diagnosis includes pneumonia, urinary tract infection, wound infection, postperfusion syndrome and postcardiotomy syndrome.

Of postcardiac surgical patients, 3.5% have a bacteremia, but only 5% of these develop prosthetic valve endocarditis. Associated laboratory findings include a normochromic anemia, a leukocytosis and an increase in the erythrocyte sedimentation rate and in C-reactive protein – these abnormalities are of course non-specific.

Patients must be reassessed carefully on a daily basis to detect early signs of deterioration or evidence of complications. Indications for early reoperation relate to either damage to the valve/valve ring or to the identity of the infecting organism. Damage to the valve/valve ring can result in increasing cardiac failure, an unstable (rocking) prosthesis, increasing valvular regurgitation or valvular obstruction. Serial echocardiography is an essential part of this continuous assessment. Increasing degrees of heart block, shown on serial electrocardiograms, suggest infection extending from the aortic valve ring into the upper part of the interventricular septum causing damage to the bundle of His. This is an uncommon indication for early surgery. Indications for early reoperation may also relate to uncontrolled infection or relapse, and, sometimes, fungal infection. Early (as opposed to late) prosthetic valve endocarditis, emboli and failure to isolate an organism are all high-risk situations and consequently are regarded by some as an indication for early reoperation.

Fungal endocarditis

Fungal infections account for less than 1% of all cases of infective endocarditis and for only 5% in intravenous drug abusers. However, these cases do present unique difficulties. It has been known for approximately 50 years that some groups of patients are at increased risk of developing this type of infection – those who have had previous cardiac surgery, patients on long-term antibiotics, patients with long-term intravenous lines, and intravenous drug abusers. These groups, however, account for less than 10% of the total. Also at risk are immunocompromised patients, including those with malignant disease and those on long-term steroids. Within the group who are at risk because of high-dose antibiotics, there is a significant number of patients being treated for bacterial endocarditis. In some reports, fungal endocarditis accounts for 10% of cases of prosthetic valve endocarditis.

Approximately 75% of all cases are caused by *Candida* spp. and most of the rest by *Aspergillus* spp. Clinical findings are similar to those of bacterial endocarditis. Particular problems with fungal endocarditis are related both to diagnosis and to treatment. Blood cultures are often negative, especially with aspergillus infection, and, furthermore, fungemia *per se* does not necessarily mean that there is endocarditis. Fungal endocarditis should be suspected in any patient from one of the high-risk groups who has culture-negative endocarditis, large vegetations (on echo-cardiography), major emboli (because fungal endocarditis produces large vegetations), and a poor response to antibiotics. Treatment is difficult because it is often impossible or impractical to remove the 'risk factor', and because therapy with medications which have a low therapeutic/toxic ratio has to be prolonged, sometimes for life.

Fungal endocarditis is often regarded as an indication for valve replacement because eradication with medication is very difficult, and because the large vegetations often cause emboli. However, there are well-documented cases of long-term control with continuous use of antifungal drugs, and in carefully selected cases this may be preferable to surgery.

Intravenous drug users

A great deal has been written about infective endocarditis in intravenous drug abusers, although it does not appear to be a major problem outside North America. Drug addicts are at increased risk of infective endocarditis because foreign material may be injected and cause endothelial trauma and because they are often immunocompromised. Additional problems are caused by the presence of other infections such as human immunodeficiency virus and hepatitis B.

Statistics regarding clinical features vary widely – 60–95% of cases involve the tricuspid valve, most of whom do not have previously documented heart disease. A significant minority do not have a heart murmur on admission. Almost two-thirds complain of chest pain and more than 50% have findings suggestive of pulmonary embolism on their initial chest X-ray – this figure subsequently rises to about 75%. Infection caused by *Staphylococcus aureus* accounts for 60–80% of cases. However, the mortality in this group of patients is low, approximately 10%. Most problems occur in those patients with large vegetations which are associated in some cases with the development of

adult respiratory distress syndrome. Surgery is advised for persistent or recurrent infection, fungal endocarditis or for when there are especially large vegetations.

Chronic renal failure

Patients with chronic renal failure are at increased risk for several reasons; a significant number are on long-term steroid therapy and many have arteriovenous fistulae or indwelling cannulae (for chronic ambulatory peritoneal dialysis).

Diagnosis is difficult because body temperature tends to be low in chronic renal failure, and therefore there is an increased likelihood that the patient will be apyrexial. Furthermore, two features – a normo-chromic anemia and bacteremia, which in other patients might lead to suspicion of a chronic infection, are both common in chronic renal failure. Consequently, unless the possibility of infective endocarditis is always considered when the patient's condition changes for no obvious cause, the diagnosis will be missed.

Infective endocarditis in the elderly

As we have seen, infective endocarditis in the elderly is becoming more common. Suggested reasons for this include immunosuppression for malignant disease, an increased use of invasive procedures and the fact that the population is, in general, living longer. One of the effects of increased longevity is that more of the population now survive to develop degenerative heart disease, such as aortic stenosis and mitral valve ring calcification. Both of these pathologies are increasingly recognized as underlying infective endocarditis. Likely sources of infection include dental and genitourinary procedures, indwelling lines and retained prosthetic materials. Problems specific to or more common in the elderly include general frailty and the fact that other pathologies are often present. It has already been noted that a toxic encephalopathy is more common in the elderly, as is a normal temperature at presentation. For all of these reasons the condition is initially incor-rectly diagnosed in up to two-thirds of elderly patients.

The mortality in older patients is twice that of younger patients, partly for the reasons given but also because staphylococcal infections are more common, which in turn predicates a higher incidence of systemic emboli. Severe coronary artery disease is more common in the elderly, which may be an additional factor.

Culture-negative endocarditis

Culture-negative endocarditis presents particular problems mainly because, in the absence of positive blood cultures, the diagnosis is likely to be either rejected or delayed. In addition, antibiotic therapy is based on an 'assumed' causative agent.

It is known that the number of organisms in blood samples varies from patient to patient (between 1 and 100/ml) but that the figure is fairly constant in any one patient – it has also been shown that the valves of patients with culture-negative endocarditis, examined microscopically following valve replacement surgery, are more often devoid of organisms than the valves from patients with positive blood cultures.

Other causes of culture negative endocarditis are:

(1) *Prior antibiotic therapy*: it has been observed that, at the time of emergency valve replacement, the damaged valve is often sterile after as little as 10 days of antibiotic treatment. Following even a short course of antibiotics, it may take 2–3 weeks for cultures again to become positive. Several studies have demonstrated an increased incidence of prior antibiotic treatment in culture-negative endocarditis compared with culture-positive cases.

(2) *The nature of the infecting organism*: this applies to rickettsiae (for example, Q fever) *Chlamydia* and infection by fastidious organisms such as *Legionella* and *Brucella*. Cases of fungal endocarditis, especially those due to filamentous fungi, are often culture-negative. Appropriate serology should always be requested in culture-negative endocarditis.

Clearly, in culture-negative cases, clinical findings, echocardiography and ancillary investigations such as levels of circulating immune complexes play a particularly important role.

Conclusion
It can be seen that, even after successful treatment of infective endocarditis, patients in each of these groups will always be in a high-risk category for further attacks.

Clinical management

Once the diagnosis has been established, a reappraisal of the patient's clinical condition should follow, bearing in mind those serious complications which demand prompt action. If clinical examination suggests cardiac failure, it should be confirmed by a chest X-ray. If not already done, echocardiography should be obtained to indicate the valve(s) affected, the state of the left ventricle and the presence of intracardiac complications (see page 27). Patients with cardiac failure should be transferred to a cardiac center where there is prompt access to open heart surgery. Some patients will be too ill to delay surgery while cardiac catheterization is carried out, but when time permits it can provide valuable information, particularly regarding coronary artery anatomy. However, not all patients with cardiac failure need an emergency operation – some can be managed medically for days or even weeks. There are obvious advantages to this delay when it is appropriate; it allows time for the patient's condition to stabilize, for infection to clear, and for the infected tissue to heal and thus make it easier to operate upon.

Cerebral signs and symptoms must always be fully assessed without delay. Focal signs and a deteriorating or changing mental state require investigation by computerized tomography to document any intracerebral pathology which may require neurosurgery (e.g. cerebral abscess), and because the findings may have an important bearing on the timing of, or suitability for, open heart surgery.

Evidence of intra-abdominal or peripheral emboli should be investigated and treated along conventional lines.

Even when the course of the disease appears uncomplicated, the natural history of infective endocarditis is such that regular re-examination and reinvestigation of the patient is essential for several reasons. First, the onset of cardiac failure is usually subacute or chronic rather than acute, evidence for which must be specifically sought. Second, emboli can occur even after suppression of the infection by antibiotics and require treatment. Furthermore, mycotic emboli may weaken the arterial wall and lead to aneurysm formation or rupture, several weeks or even months later (see pages 23 and 34). Third, renal failure may develop insidiously.

Echocardiography should be repeated weekly in native valve endocarditis unless the clinical condition requires it sooner. Follow-up may be needed more often for prosthetic valve endocarditis. A full blood count and urea and electrolytes should be checked every few days. Patients with tricuspid endocarditis must have regular chest X-rays, plus V/Q scans when indicated.

Patients whose antibiotic regimen includes an aminoglycoside or vancomycin need to have pre- and postdose antibiotic levels monitored regularly. The aminoglycosides (usually gentamicin or netilmicin) cause dose-related auditory and vestibular VIIIth nerve damage. An early sign of auditory damage is tinnitus and of vestibular damage, movement-related headache, dizziness, and nausea. These symptoms require cessation or reduction of the drug. Dose-related renal damage is well documented and is especially likely in the presence of hypotension, in the elderly, and with loop diuretics. Vancomycin causes dose-related auditory damage in the form of tinnitus and deafness. Nephrotoxicity can also occur.

Persistence or recrudescence of fever during treatment is quite common. There are several possible causes. The most likely is the presence of extensive infection of the valve ring. This is more common with aortic than with mitral valve endocarditis. If repeat echocardiography (preferably transesophageal) demonstrates this, then surgery is usually advised. Other causes are systemic or pulmonary emboli and drug hypersensitivity. In the latter situation, there is usually a generalized erythematous rash and there may be an eosinophilia with neutropenia. A change of antibiotics is then necessary. The temptation to 'blame' an infected intravenous line should be resisted as this is rarely the cause of persistent pyrexia.

Antibiotics should usually be given for 4–6 weeks. Some patients, for example, those infected with sensitive strains of viridans streptococci, may complete their course of antibiotics at home with oral medication. However, they need to attend the ward at least weekly for reassessment.

A full reassessment should be made approximately 7–10 days after cessation of antibiotics. This should include full blood count, C-reactive protein and a check on renal function. Temperature should be checked and blood cultures repeated.

A patient who has had an episode of infective endocarditis has a risk of further attacks comparable to that of patients with prosthetic valves. They should be advised accordingly with respect to antibiotic prophylaxis.

Late deaths

As many as 25% of patients who leave hospital, apparently cured of infective endocarditis, subsequently die from its effects during the next 10 years. Most of these late deaths are related to aortic valve endocarditis and are the result of cardiac failure secondary to severe valvular damage. Many of these deaths could, of course, be prevented by valve replacement. In some cases, the cardiac failure is acute in onset due to valve cusp rupture which can occur many months or years after the original infection. Rupture of an aortic aneurysm is another important cause of late death and may be related to infection of the aortic valve (native or prosthetic) or of coarctation of the aorta. The implications of these observations are clear – all patients with infective endocarditis should be carefully reviewed after discharge from hospital, looking especially for evidence of cardiac failure. Echocardiography is also an essential part of the follow-up, in order to detect early signs of a developing aneurysm so that rupture can be pre-empted by surgery.

Late recurrence or recrudescence of infection occurs in about 5% of cases. Diagnosis may be especially difficult in this situation because blood cultures may be negative (see above) and because echocardiography will probably show persistence of the previous vegetations. In these cases, estimation of C-reactive protein and of immune complexes may be helpful – especially if baseline levels were measured prior to discharge following the original infection.

Section 2   Infective Endocarditis Illustrated

List of illustrations

Figure 1
Non-bacterial thrombotic endocarditis. Vegetations on the mitral valve of an elderly lady who died from carcinoma of the gallbladder

Figure 2
Non-bacterial thrombotic endocarditis on aortic valve

Figure 3
Non-bacterial thrombotic endocarditis on tricuspid valve

Figure 4
A normal aortic valve

Figure 5
A normal mitral valve

Figure 6
A floppy mitral valve showing redundant cusp tissue (mitral valve prolapse)

Figure 7
Degenerative aortic stenosis

Figure 8
A stenosed bicuspid aortic valve

Figure 9
Osteomyelitis (Brodie's abscess)

Figure 10
Sinusitis

Figure 11
An eroded infected pacemaker

Figure 12
Severe dental caries

Figure 13
Acute aortic valve endocarditis

Figure 14
Mitral valve vegetations

Figure 15
Microscopy showing *Staphylococcus aureus* aortic valve endocarditis

Figure 16
Aortic valve endocarditis

Figure 17
Mitral valve chordae tendineae

Figure 18
Intracardiac pressure tracings in a patient with severe acute mitral regurgitation

Figure 19
Chest X-ray showing acute pulmonary edema

Figure 20
Chest X-ray showing a 60-year-old female patient with staphylococcal aortic valve endocarditis

Figure 21
Cerebral embolism

Figure 22
Computerized tomography scan of brain showing a dark area of low attenuation in the frontoparietal region

Figure 23
Computerized tomography scan of brain showing a high attenuation white area in the frontoparietal region

Figure 24
Computerized tomography scan of brain showing an intracerebral (occipital) abscess

Figure 25
Small subcapsular splenic infarction

Figure 26
Abdominal ultrasound showing two areas of splenic infarction

Figure 27
Focal glomerulonephritis showing the usual lobular architecture

Figure 28
Renal infarction

Figure 29
DMSA renal scan posterior view

Figure 30
DMSA renal scan anterior view

Figure 31
Purpura

Figure 32
Finger clubbing

Figure 33
Subconjunctival hemorrhage

Figure 34
Splinter hemorrhages and finger clubbing

Figure 35
Splinter hemorrhages

Figure 36
Osler node

Figure 37
Janeway lesion

Figure 38
Roth spots

Figure 39
Libman–Sacks endocarditis

Figure 40
Acute rheumatic carditis

Figure 41
M-mode echocardiogram showing typical appearances of left atrial myxoma

Figure 42
Transthoracic echocardiography of the normal heart, viewed from the front

Figure 43
Schematic representation of the heart as viewed from behind

Figure 44
Transesophageal echocardiography of the normal heart

Figure 45
Transthoracic echocardiography – parasternal long-axis view showing abnormal echoes in the root of the aorta

Figure 46
Transesophageal echocardiography of the same patient as shown in Figure 45, showing a mass at the aortic valve orifice

Figure 47
Operative findings on the same patient as shown in Figures 45 and 46 viewed from above, showing a large vegetation attached to the aortic valve

Figure 48
Transthoracic echocardiography showing apical four-chamber view in a patient with mitral valve endocarditis

Figure 49
Transesophageal echocardiography in the same patient as shown in Figure 48. An abnormal mass is seen attached to both mitral valve cusps

Figure 50
Transthoracic echocardiography – parasternal long-axis view, showing a very abnormal mitral valve

Figure 51
Transesophageal echocardiography in same patient as shown in Figure 50, showing the prosthetic mitral valve with no vegetations

Figure 52
M-mode echocardiography of mitral valve. Echoes behind the valve are suspicious of left atrial myxoma

Figure 53
Transthoracic echocardiography – parasternal long-axis view. There is no evidence of tumor in the left atrium, but it is obviously an abnormal mitral valve

Figure 54
Left ventriculogram showing severe paravalvar mitral regurgitation

Figure 55

Aortogram showing severe aortic regurgitation of aortic bioprosthesis

Figure 56

Aortogram showing severe aortic regurgitation and vegetations

Figure 57

Left coronary angiogram

Figure 58

Transesophageal echocardiography showing infective endocarditis involving a prosthetic aortic valve

Figure 59

α-Hemolytic streptococcus showing greening of the blood agar culture medium

Figure 60

α-Hemolytic streptococcus on blood agar showing the inhibition of growth round the antibiotic-containing discs

Figure 61

A culture of *Streptococcus bovis* biotype I on blood agar together with API 20 streptococcus test used in identification

Figure 62

Test-tube method of estimating the minimum inhibitory concentration and minimum bactericidal concentration

Figure 63

Demonstration of bactericidal synergy between benzylpenicillin and netilmicin by a layer-plate technique

Figure 64

Colonies of *Staphylococcus aureus* growing on blood agar

Figure 65

Identification of coagulase-positive staphylococci

Figure 66

Penicillin-resistant *Staphylococcus aureus* showing susceptibility to fucidin, erythromycin, rifampicin, gentamicin and vancomycin

Figure 67

Determination of flucloxacillin susceptibility

Figure 68

Pseudomonas aeruginosa growing on nutrient agar

and showing development of green pigment by the bacterial colonies

Figure 69

Assembly of all the required equipment for venepuncture

Figure 70

Thorough washing of the hands prior to venepuncture

Figure 71

Venepuncture using the 'no-touch' technique, after the venepuncture site has been disinfected

Figure 72

Needle change prior to inoculation of culture bottles

Figure 73

Addition of the recommended volume of blood to aerobic and anaerobic culture bottles

Figure 74

Lateral chest X-ray showing three prosthetic heart valves (tricuspid, aortic and mitral)

Figure 75

Starr Edwards aortic valve prosthesis

Figure 76

Prosthetic valve endocarditis

Figure 77

Transthoracic echocardiography – left parasternal long-axis view. The mitral valve is irregularly thickened with a mass protruding into the left atrium

Figure 78

Same patient as shown in Figure 77 – right parasternal short-axis view

Figure 79

Same patient as shown in Figures 77 and 78. Valves as seen at postmortem examination

Figure 80

Fungal infection of a prosthetic valve (*Aspergillus* spp.)

Figure 81

Microscopy of valve tissue from the same patient as shown in Figure 80. The fungi are stained black

Figure 82

Tricuspid valve vegetations

Figure 83

Right ventriculogram showing severe tricuspid regurgitation due to tricuspid endocarditis

Figure 84
Transthoracic echocardiography – four-chamber view, showing large vegetation on the tricuspid valve
Figure 85
Chest X-ray showing lung abscesses
Figure 86
Chest X-ray showing radiological findings consistent with pulmonary embolism
Figure 87
V/Q scan showing marked ventilation perfusion mismatch
Figure 88
Aortic valve endocarditis caused by *Chlamydia psittaci* (psittacosis)
Figure 89
Microscopy of the valve shown in Figure 88 using Machieavello stain
Figure 90
Maculopapular rash caused by penicillin allergy in a patient with prosthetic valve endocarditis
Figure 91
Benign villous adenoma (polyp) of colon
Figure 92
Barium enema showing filling defects due to carcinoma of the ascending colon

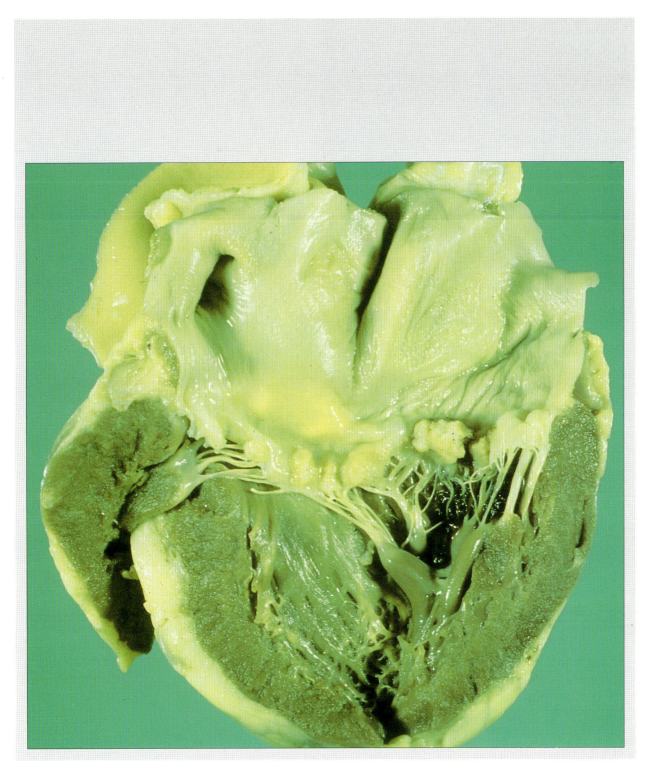

Figure 1   Non-bacterial thrombotic endocarditis. Vegetations on the mitral valve of an elderly lady who died from carcinoma of the gallbladder. Other conditions associated with non-bacterial thrombotic endocarditis are disseminated intervascular coagulation and hemodialysis

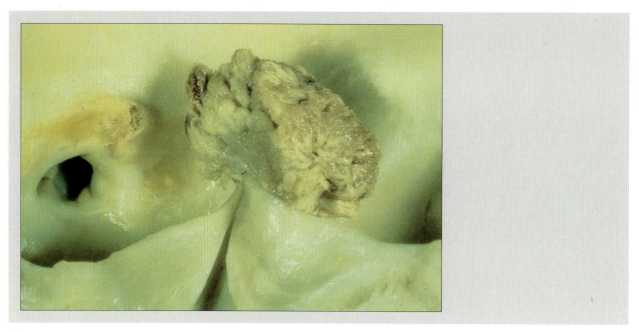

Figure 2 Non-bacterial thrombotic endocarditis on aortic valve

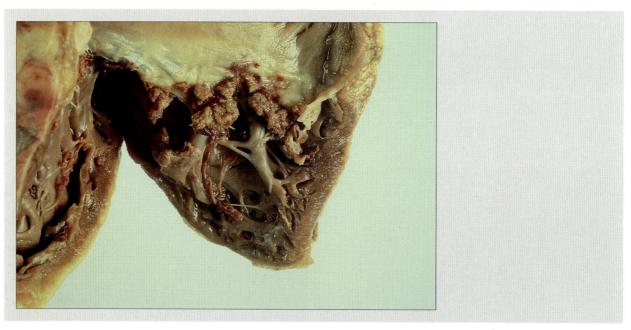

Figure 3 Non-bacterial thrombotic endocarditis on tricuspid valve. Non-bacterial thrombotic endocarditis had been described in 1%–2% of routine postmortem examinations. It results from the deposition of platelets and fibrin at sites of microscopic endothelial trauma which is especially common in congenital and acquired valvular defects. Bacteria adhere to and colonize these lesions which are now regarded as the common precursor of infective endocarditis

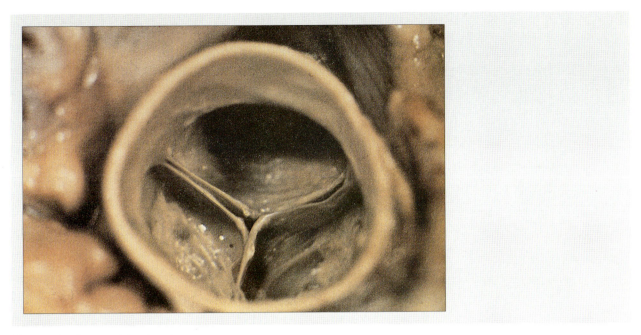

Figure 4 A normal aortic valve

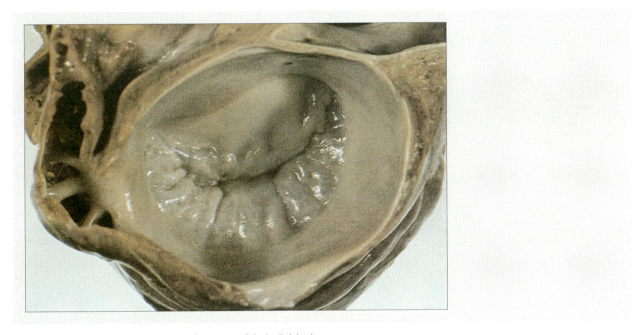

Figure 5 A normal mitral valve. In susceptible individuals non-bacterial thrombotic endocarditis may form on normal valves

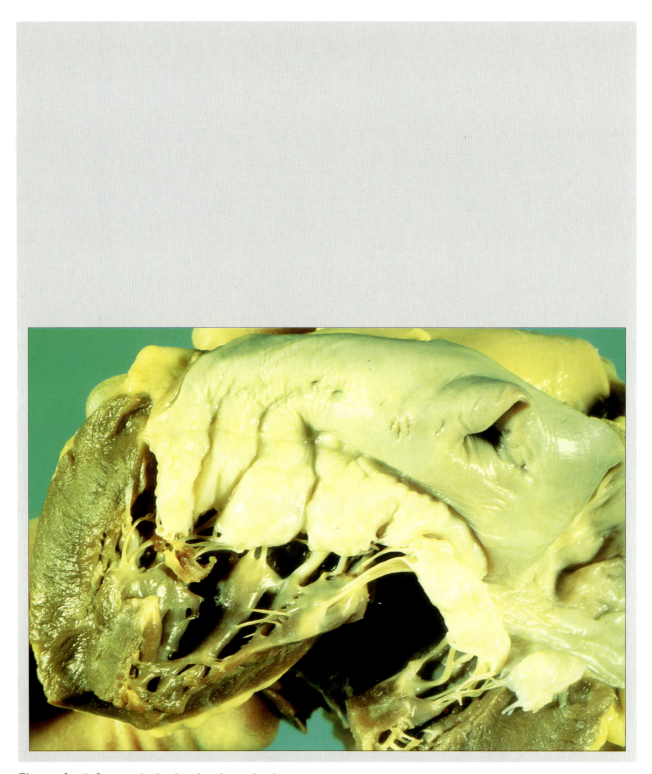

Figure 6 A floppy mitral valve showing redundant cusp tissue (mitral valve prolapse). This is now one of the commonest substrates for infective endocarditis

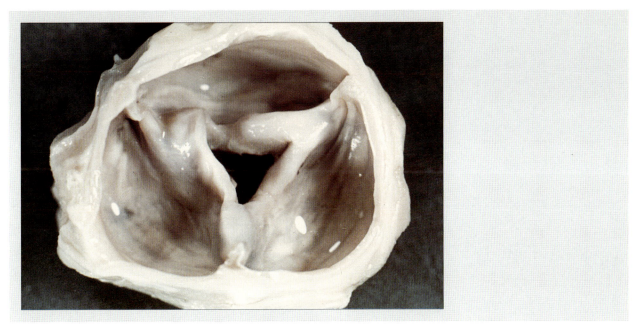

Figure 7 Degenerative aortic stenosis. Elderly patients with degenerative aortic valve disease are increasingly recognized as a high-risk group for infective endocarditis

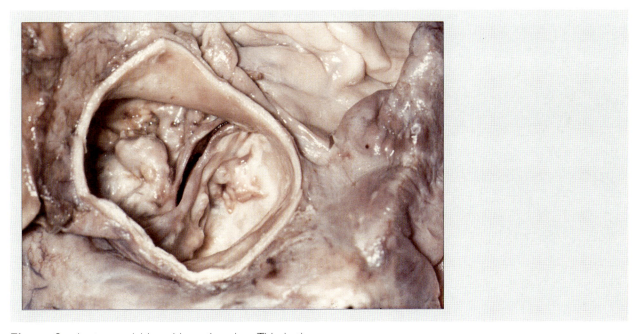

Figure 8 A stenosed bicuspid aortic valve. This is the commonest congenital valvular defect and is often unrecognized until an episode of infective endocarditis

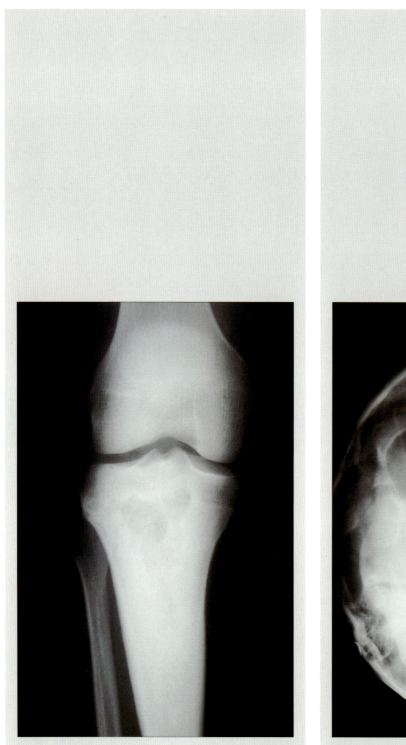

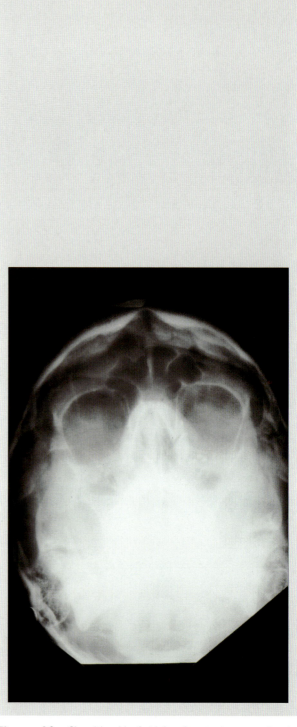

Figure 9 Osteomyelitis (Brodie's abscess). The possibility of infective endocarditis should be considered in any patient with a heart murmur and osteomyelitis. At one time this was a common association

Figure 10 Sinusitis. Air fluid levels can be seen in the frontal sinuses. Any form of infection which is associated with intermittent bacteremia is a potential cause of infective endocarditis. Every effort should be made to eradicate such foci in susceptible patients

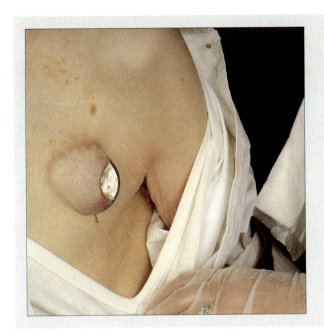

Figure 11   An eroded infected pacemaker. This is an uncommon but well-recognized cause of infective endocarditis, usually of the tricuspid valve. Although antibiotic prophylaxis is normally given at the time of pacemaker implantation it does not prevent endocarditis occurring in this situation since erosion often occurs weeks or months after pacemaker implantation

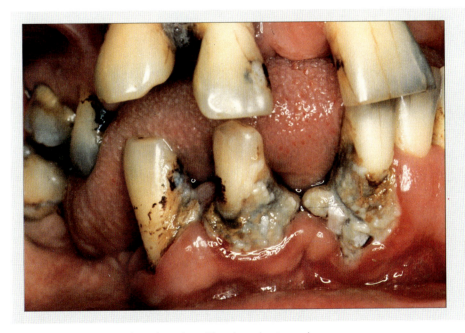

Figure 12   Severe dental caries. Transient bacteremia occurs with dental extraction and periodontal surgery. Spontaneous bacteremia occurs in the presence of severe periodontal disease

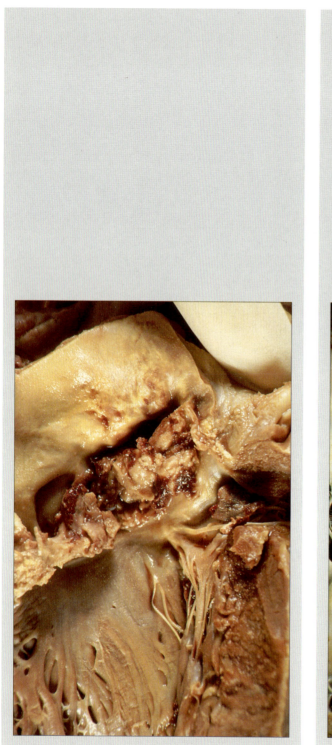

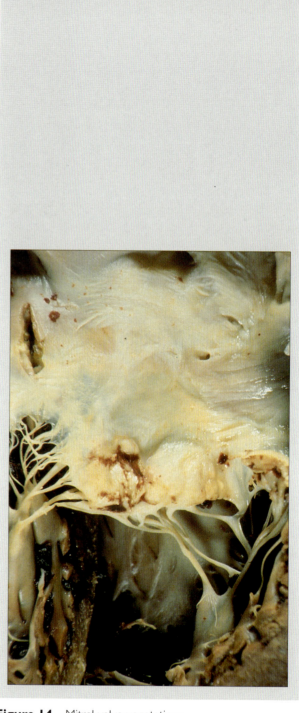

Figure 13 Acute aortic valve endocarditis caused by *Staphylococcus aureus*. Vegetations caused by this organism are characteristically large and friable which results in a high incidence of emboli

Figure 14 Mitral valve vegetations

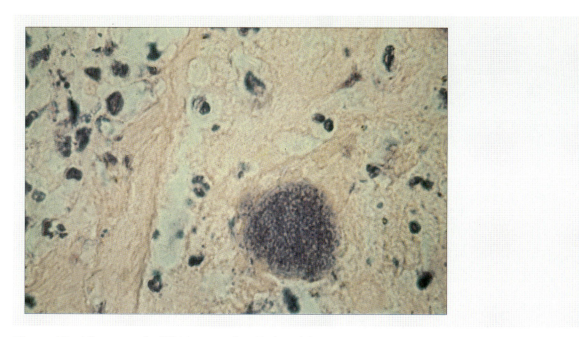

Figure 15 Microscopy (× 400 Hematoxylin – Eosin stain). *Staphylococcus aureus* aortic valve endocarditis showing a large clump of organisms

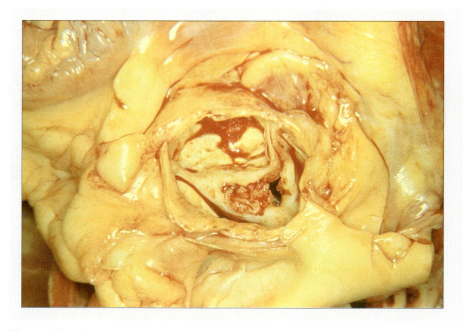

Figure 16 Aortic valve endocarditis. This is a congenitally bicuspid valve. A vegetation is clearly seen on the lower cusp where it has caused a perforation. This led to rapidly fatal left ventricular failure

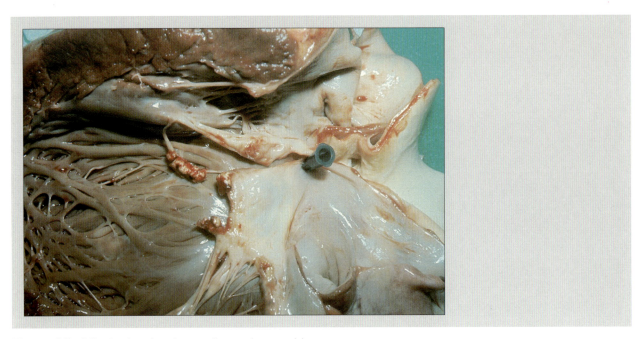

Figure 17 Mitral valve chordae tendineae destroyed by staphylococcal endocarditis. This is another important cause of sudden left ventricular failure

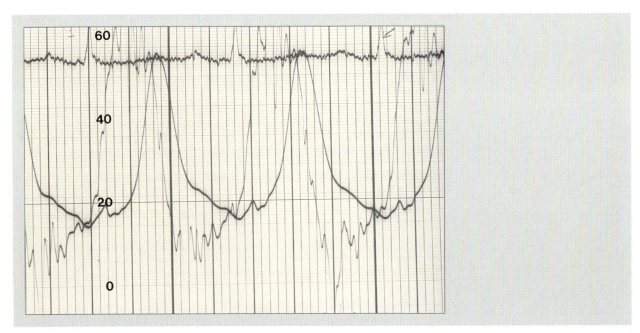

Figure 18 Intracardiac pressure tracings in a patient with severe acute mitral regurgitation. Simultaneous left ventricular and indirect left atrial (wedge) pressures. The peak left ventricular and left atrial pressures equalize before the end of systole. When this happens, the murmur stops. Thus, sometimes, only a short early systolic murmur is heard despite severe mitral regurgitation

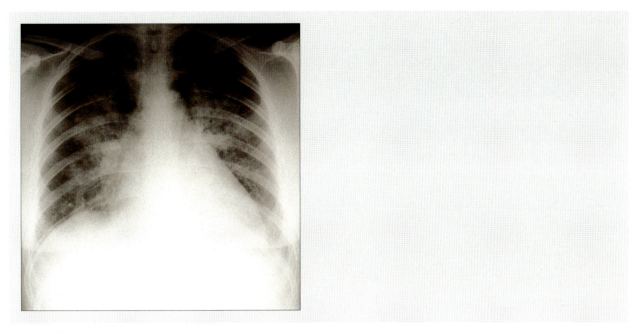

Figure 19 Chest X-ray. Acute pulmonary edema. In a patient with infective endocarditis this usually is the result of severe valvular damage and is responsible for almost two-thirds of all deaths. Valve replacement is indicated often as an emergency procedure

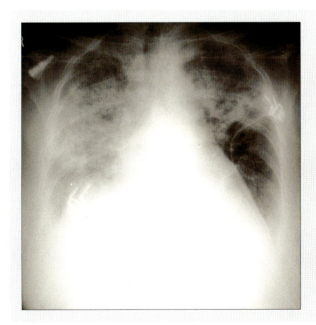

Figure 20 Chest X-ray. Sixty-year-old female patient with staphylococcal aortic valve endocarditis. The X-ray appearances were initially attributed to pulmonary edema. However, indirect left atrial pressure was normal and blood gas analysis showed severe arterial hypoxemia. The correct diagnosis is adult respiratory distress syndrome. This resolved with antibiotics and was followed by successful aortic valve replacement

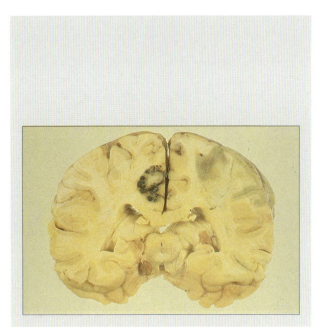

Figure 21 Cerebral embolism. This is a major cause of death in infective endocarditis and is especially common in acute as opposed to subacute cases. Computerized tomography distinguishes between infarction, hemorrhage and abscess and should be performed in all patients with focal neurological signs

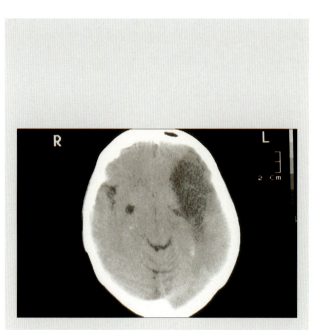

Figure 22 Computerized tomography scan of brain showing a dark area of low attenuation in the frontoparietal region. This indicates cerebral infarction

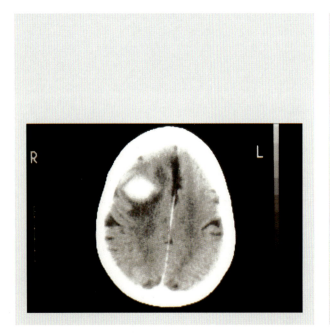

Figure 23 Computerized tomography scan of brain showing a high attenuation white area in the frontoparietal region. This indicates cerebral hemorrhage

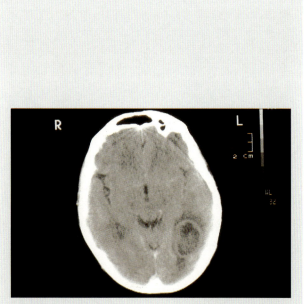

Figure 24 Computerized tomography scan of brain showing an intracerebral (occipital) abscess. The lesion has a dark center surrounded by a pale periphery. Focal neurological signs must be investigated promptly to distinguish between hemorrhage, infarction and abcess so that treatment is appropriate. An intracerebral hemorrage is a contraindication to open-heart surgery because further bleeding will occur when the patient is anticoagulated

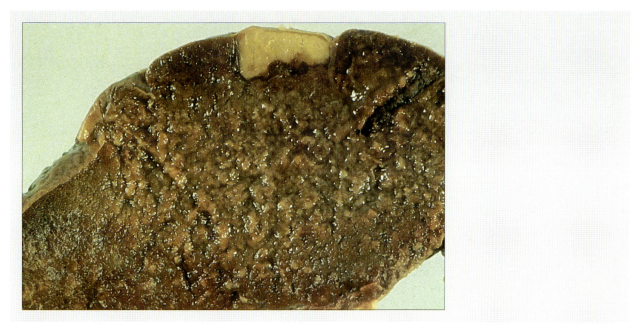

Figure 25 Small subcapsular splenic infarction. Sixty-four-year-old female patient with disseminated carcinoma of the colon who died from acute aortic valve infective endocarditis

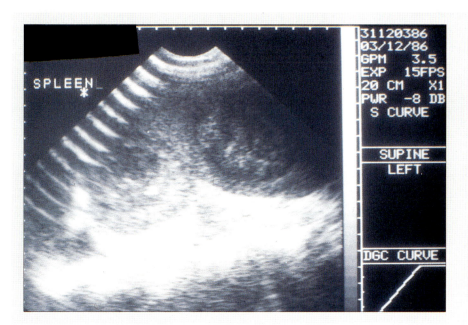

Figure 26 Abdominal ultrasound. Two areas of splenic infarction are shown. These were the results of emboli from an infected mitral valve. Many splenic emboli are silent but typically abdominal pain and pleuritic left shoulder tip pain occur. Ultrasound does not distinguish sterile infarction from an embolic abscess. If the latter is suspected, computerized tomography will make the distinction

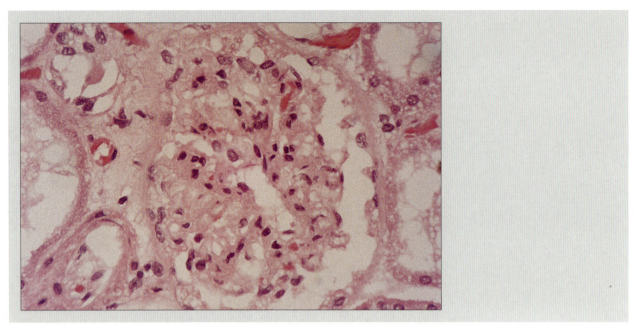

Figure 27 Focal glomerulonephritis showing the usual lobular architecture. There is some evidence of tuft adhesions on the left hand side. This is common in infective endocarditis and is usually benign

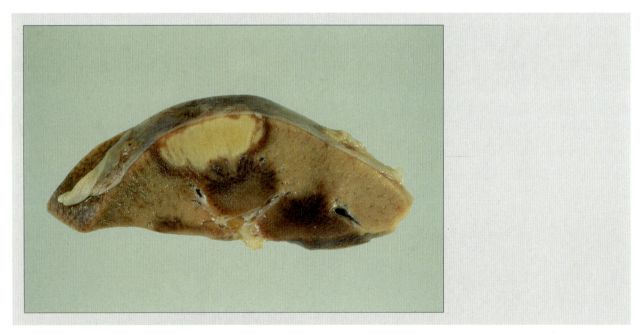

Figure 28 Renal infarction. The patient died as a result of prosthetic valve endocarditis. Renal infarction may produce loin pain association with hematuria, or silent hematuria

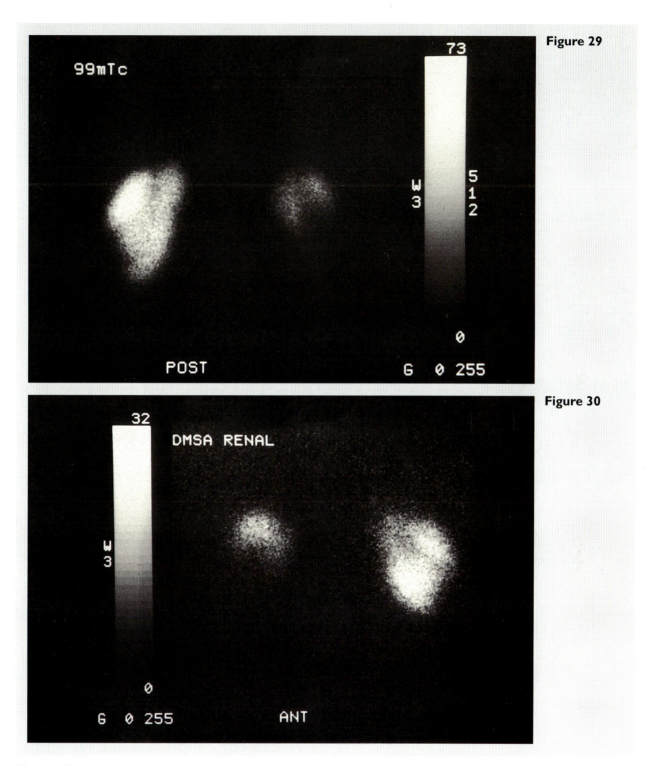

Figure 29

Figure 30

Figures 29 and 30 DMSA. Renal scan. 99m-Tc. The right kidney in Figure 29 is represented only by a crescent of functioning parenchyma at the upper pole. The left kidney in Figure 30 is on the right and is very irregular with several cortical defects. These appearances are consistent with multiple renal infarctions. The patient has had recurrent episodes of infective endocarditis. There is now evidence of progressive deterioration in renal function

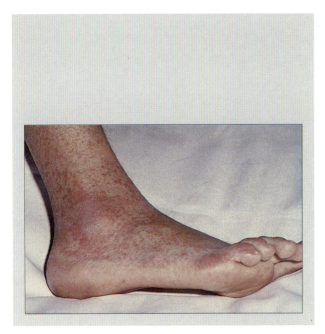

Figure 31 Purpura. Petechiae occur on the limbs and mucus membranes. Other causes include hematological disorders, vasculitis, renal failure and scurvy

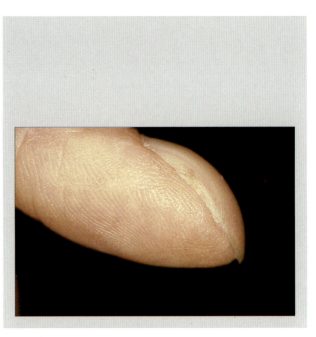

Figure 32 Finger clubbing. Other causes include carcinoma of the bronchus, suppurative lung disease and hepatic cirrhosis

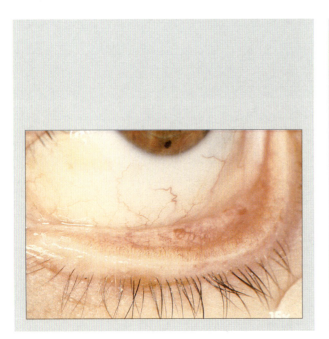

Figure 33 Subconjunctival hemorrhage

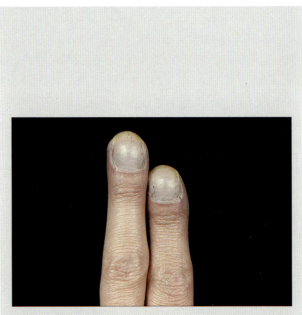

Figure 34 Splinter hemorrhages and finger clubbing. However, in this case the latter is due to cyanotic congenital heart disease – note the cyanosis. Infective endocarditis was related to a patent ductus in a patient with Eisenmenger complex

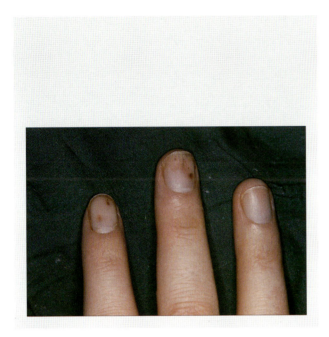

Figure 35 Splinter hemorrhages. The differential diagnosis includes trauma, brachial artery embolus, rheumatoid arthritis and trichinosis

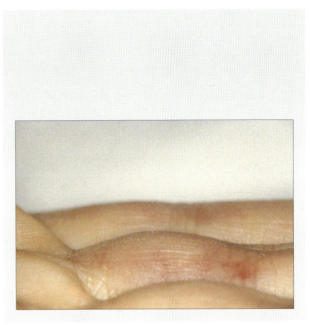

Figure 36 Osler node. These are reddened, tender swellings which last for a few hours to a few days. They may also occur in systemic lupus erythematosus, non-bacterial thrombotic endocarditis, typhoid and disseminated gonococcal infections

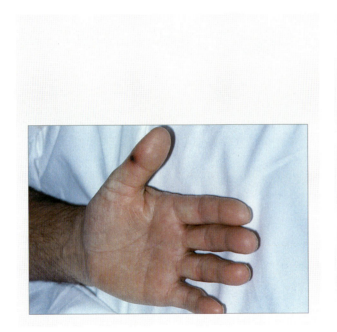

Figure 37 Janeway lesion. These are flattened, non-tender lesions, usually on the palm or sole of the foot

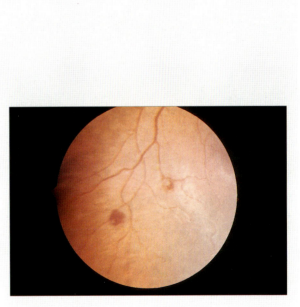

Figure 38 Roth spots. The lesions have a pale center and a red periphery

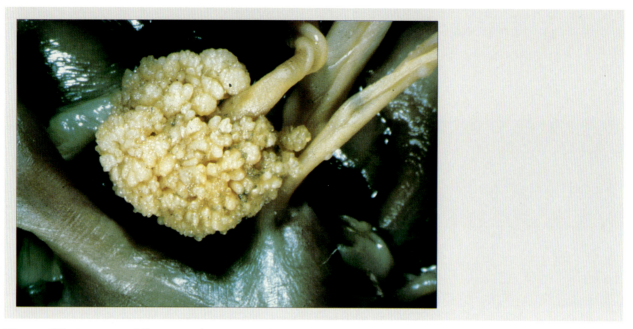

Figure 39 Large coral-like vegetations on a tricuspid valve. This is Libman–Sacks endocarditis (systemic lupus erythematosus). This condition can produce a clinical syndrome very suggestive of infective endocarditis

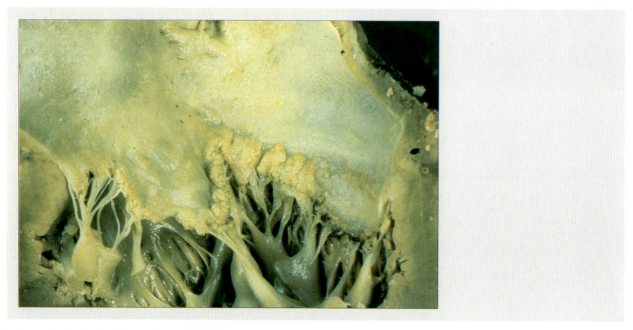

Figure 40 Acute rheumatic carditis. Verrucous vegetations on the posterior cusp of the mitral valve. The end result of this valvulitis was at one time the commonest underlying lesion in infective endocarditis

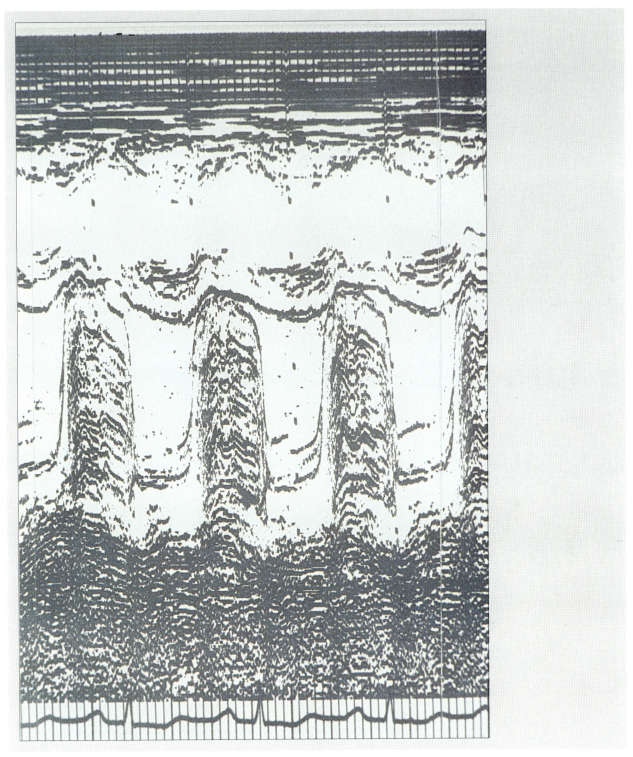

Figure 41 M-mode echocardiogram. Typical appearances of left atrial myxoma showing multiple echoes behind the mitral valve, i.e. in the left atrium. Each of the conditions shown in Figures 39, 40 and 41 (Libman–Sacks endocarditis, acute rheumatic carditis and left atrial myxoma, respectively) can produce a clinical syndrome very suggestive of infective endocarditis

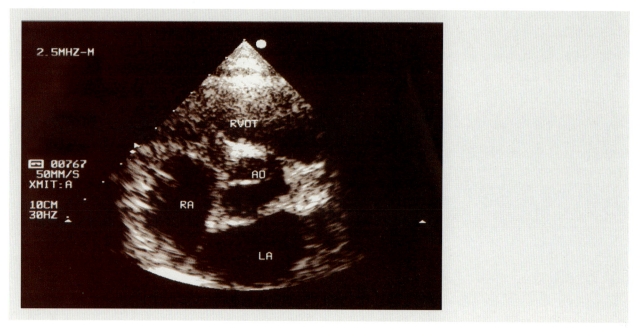

Figure 42 Transthoracic echocardiography – normal study. Conventional echocardiography views the heart from the front. The left atrium is at the bottom of the tracing as it is further away from the probe than are the other cardiac structures

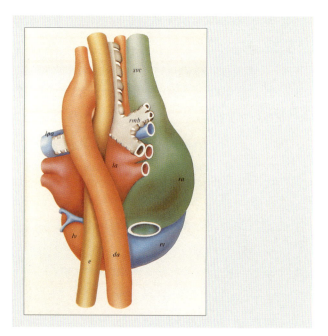

Figure 43 Schematic representation of the heart as viewed from behind. Transesophageal echocardiography is performed by passing a transducer into the esophagus and siting it behind the heart. This ensures that the transducer is closer to the heart than with conventional transthoracic echocardiography; the sound waves are thus less attenuated, a higher frequency beam can be used and this produces images of higher resolution. svc, superior vena cava; la, left atrium; ra, right atrium; rv, right ventricle; lv, left ventricle; rmb, right main bronchus; e, esophagus; da, descending aorta; lpa, left pulmonary artery

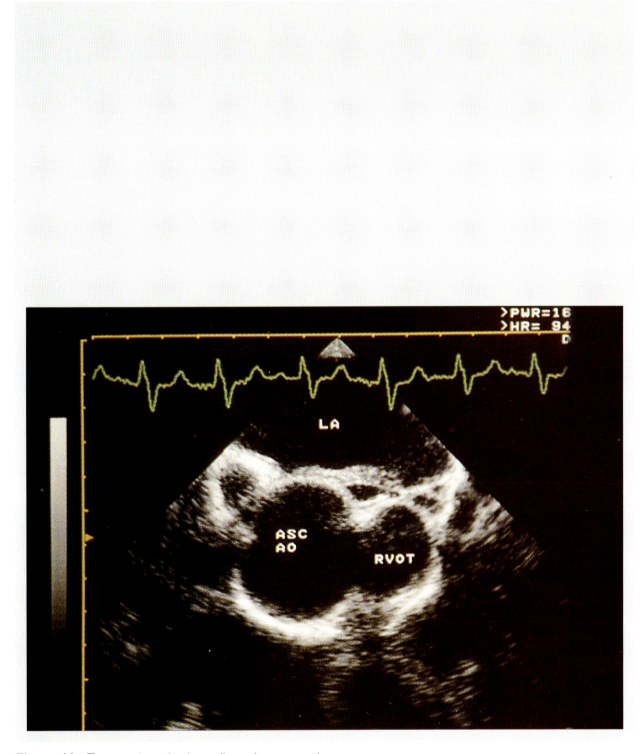

Figure 44 Transesophageal echocardiography – normal study. Note that the left atrium, being closer to the probe, is at the top of the picture (compared with Figure 42). The picture quality is better than in Figure 42

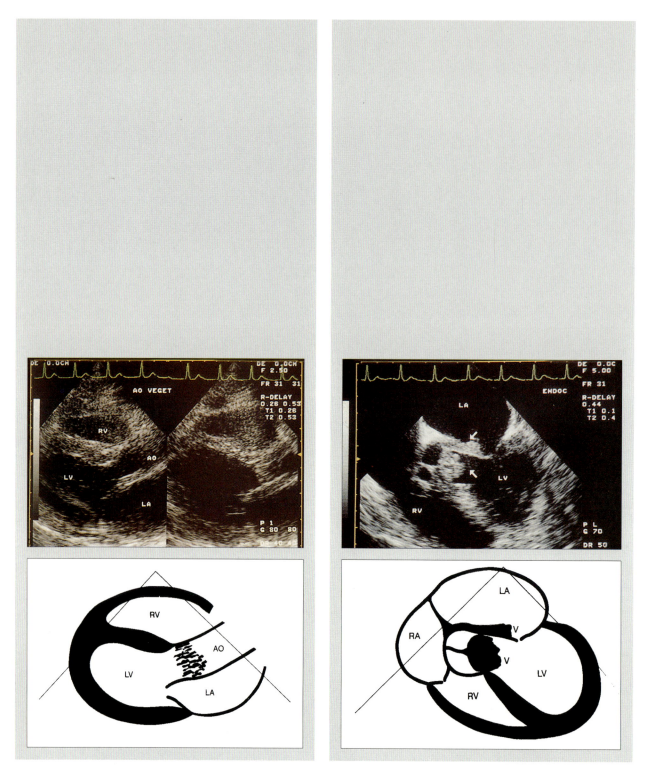

Figure 45 Transthoracic echocardiography – parasternal long-axis view. Abnormal echoes in the root of the aorta are suggestive but not diagnostic of infective endocarditis

Figure 46 Transesophageal echocardiography – same patient as shown in Figure 45. A mass is clearly seen at the aortic valve orifice. This confirms the presence of aortic valve vegetations. Vegetations are also seen on the mitral valve

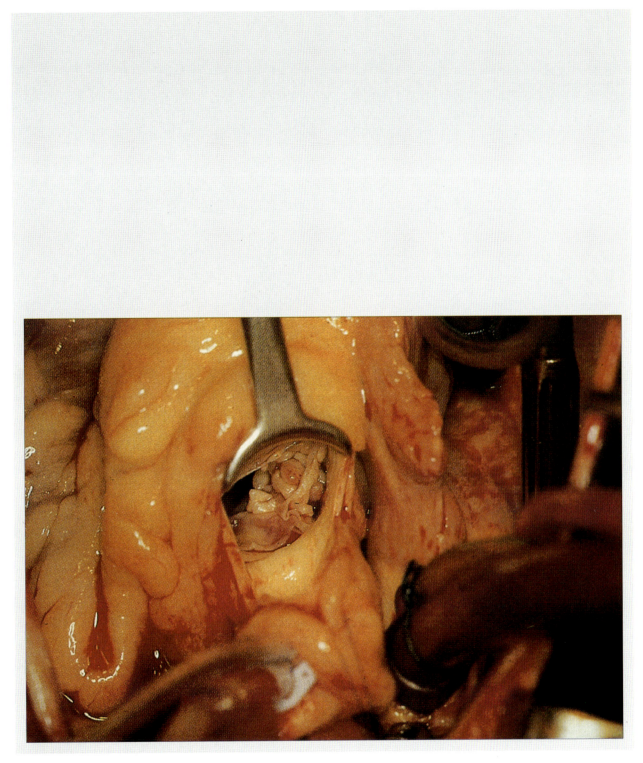

Figure 47 Operative findings in the same patient as shown in Figures 45 and 46. Viewed from above, a large vegetation is seen attached to the aortic valve

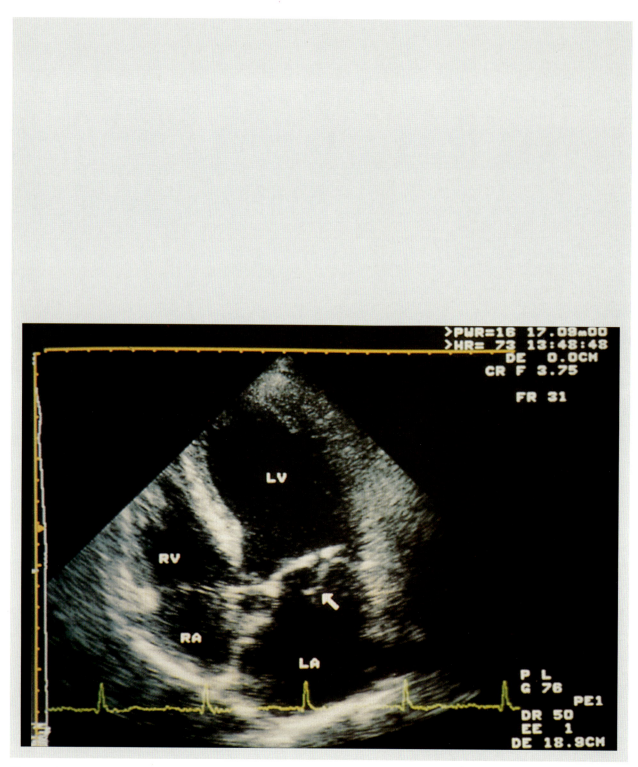

Figure 48 Transthoracic echocardiography – apical four-chamber view in a patient with mitral valve endocarditis. Arrow indicates possible mitral valve vegetation

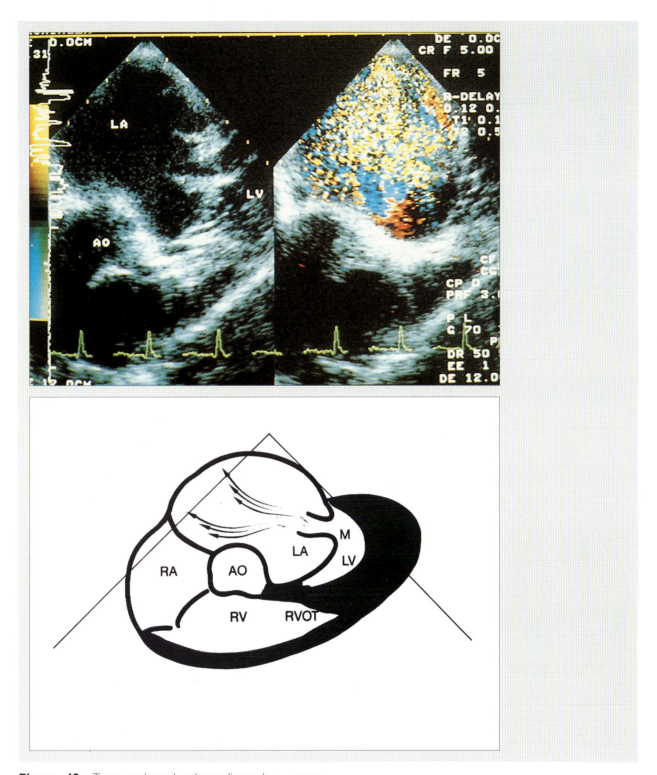

Figure 49 Transesophageal echocardiography – same patient as shown in Figure 48. Abnormal mass seen clearly attached to both mitral valve cusps. In addition, color flow Doppler tracing indicates severe turbulent mitral regurgitation which was caused by ruptured chordae tendineae

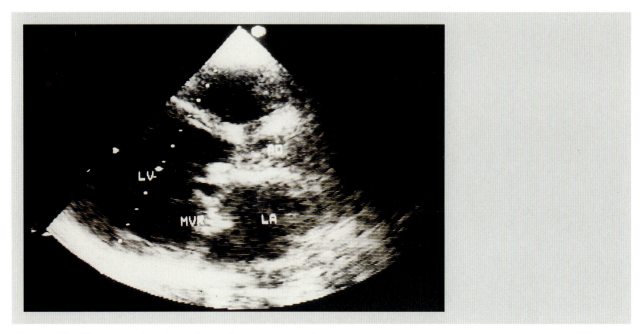

Figure 50 Transthoracic echocardiography – parasternal long-axis view. This is clearly a very abnormal mitral valve. The patient had had mitral valve replacement and suspected infective endocarditis

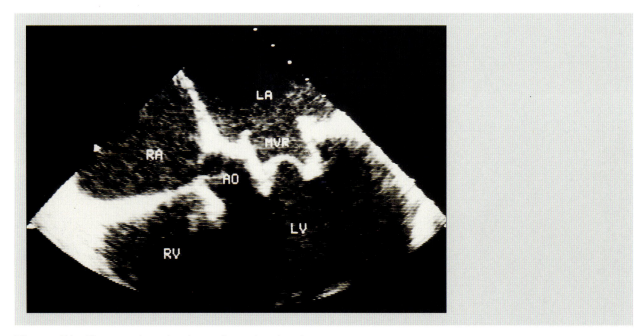

Figure 51 Transesophageal echocardiography showing that the valve shown in Figure 50 is a prosthetic mitral valve with no vegetations although this in itself does not exclude infective endocarditis. Transesophageal echocardiography should probably be performed in all cases of suspected prosthetic valve endocarditis

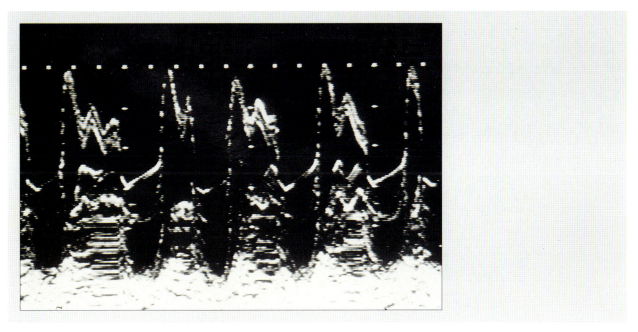

Figure 52 M-mode echocardiography of mitral valve. Echoes behind the valve are suspicious of left atrial myxoma

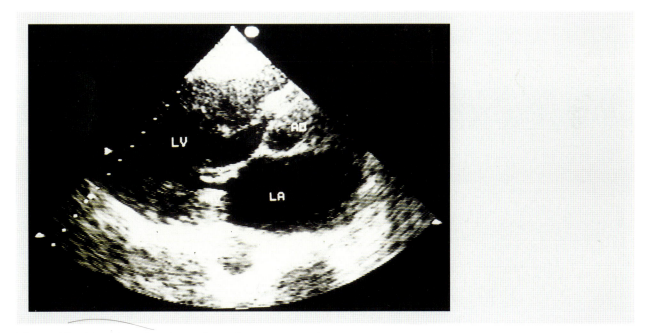

Figure 53 Transthoracic echocardiography – parasternal long-axis view. No evidence of tumor in the left atrium but obviously an abnormal mitral valve (this is due to a flail cusp). M-mode echocardiography in most situations, provides less useful information than does transthoracic echocardiography

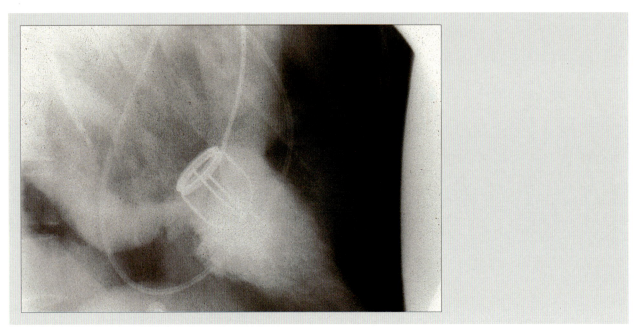

Figure 54 Left ventriculogram. Severe paravalvar mitral regurgitation. Dye can be seen sweeping around the margins of the enlarged left atrium. Paravalvar regurgitation is characteristic of prosthetic valve endocarditis because the infection is sited in the sewing ring of the valve

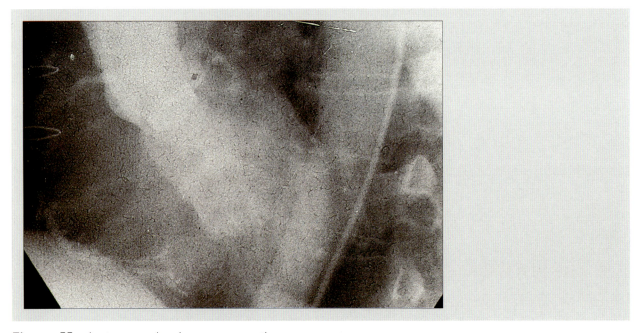

Figure 55 Aortogram showing severe aortic regurgitation. This valve is a bioprosthesis – note the stainless steel sewing ring to which the valve cusps are attached. When endocarditis involves a bioprosthesis the valve cusp may be infected in addition to infection of the valve ring

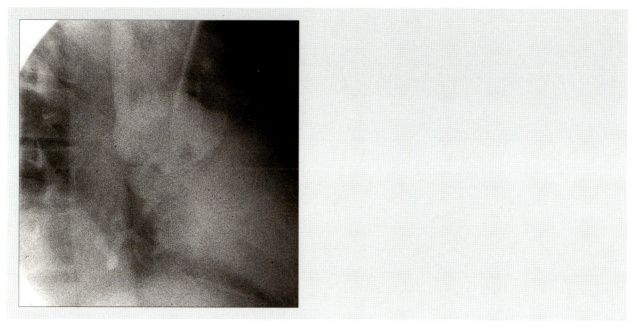

Figure 56 Aortogram. The catheter is sited in the root of the aorta. Severe aortic regurgitation is clearly seen. Note also the filling defect in the root of the aorta. This defect is due to a vegetation, an appearance not often seen at angiography

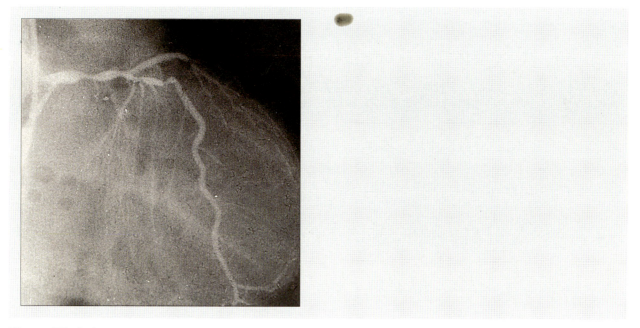

Figure 57 Left coronary angiogram. There are stenoses in the left main stem and in the left anterior descending branch. In the investigation of infective endocarditis, echocardiography has largely replaced angiography. However, the latter is still required to demonstrate the coronary artery anatomy

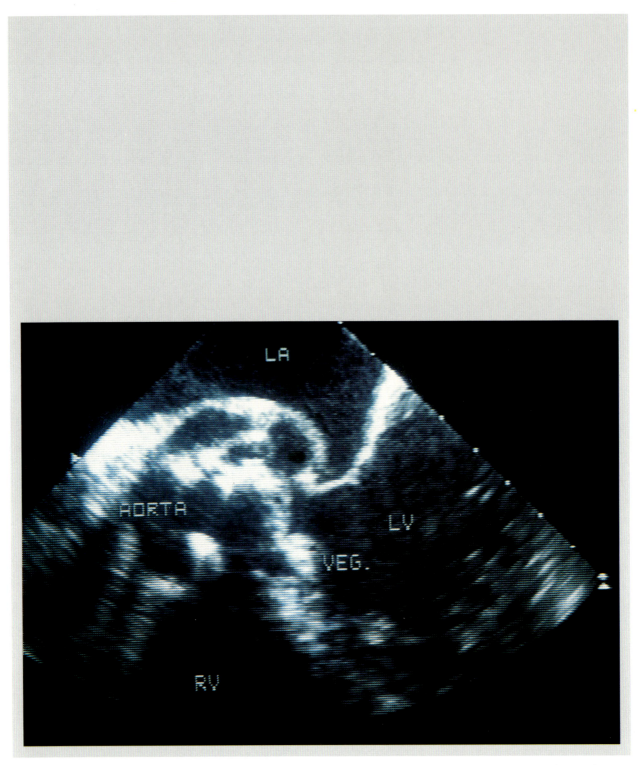

Figure 58 Transesophageal echocardiography showing infective endocarditis involving a prosthetic aortic valve. Vegetations seen prolapsing into left ventricle. Filling defects are present in the root of the aorta, between the aorta and the left atrium, and indicate a paravalvular abscess. In contrast to angiography, transesophageal echocardiography can demonstrate 80% of abscesses

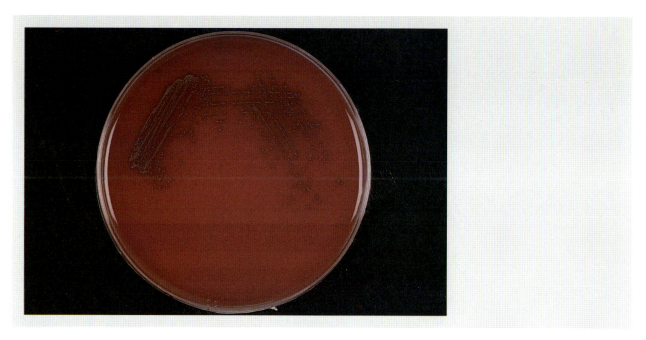

Figure 59 α-Hemolytic streptococcus showing greening of the blood agar culture medium

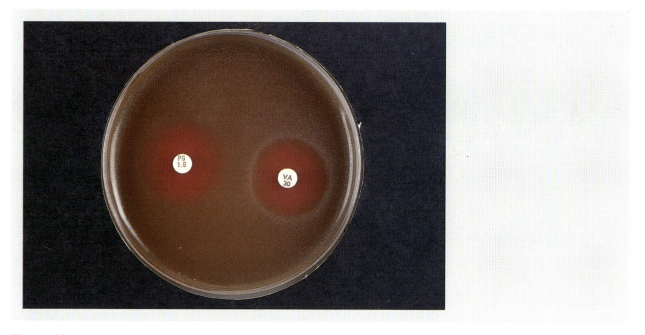

Figure 60 α-Hemolytic streptococcus on blood agar. The inhibition of growth round the antibiotic-containing discs demonstrates susceptibility to benzylpenicillin (PG 1.5) and vancomycin (VA 30)

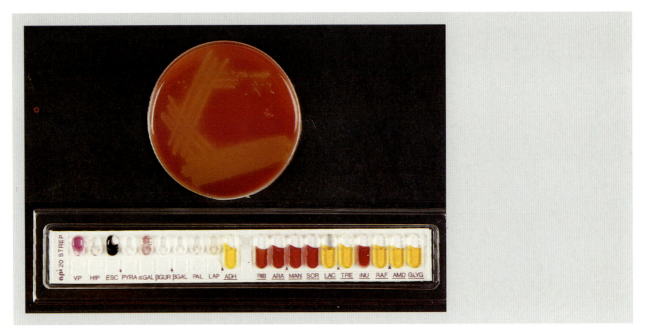

Figure 61   A culture of *Streptococcus bovis* biotype 1 on blood agar together with the API 20 streptococcus test used in identification. A suspension of the organism has been inoculated into microtubes that contain standardized substrates. Enzymatic activity or fermentation of sugars results in color changes of the media which enables identification of the isolate

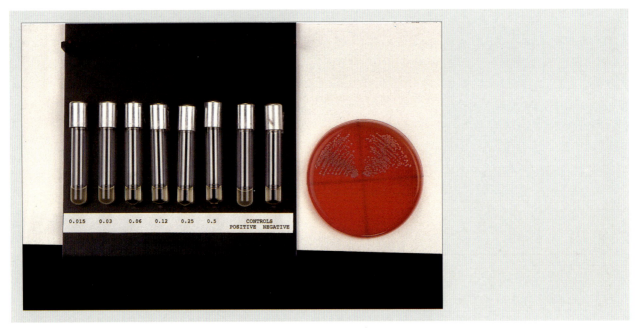

Figure 62   Test-tube method of estimating the minimum inhibitory concentration and minimum bactericidal concentration. The organism is inoculated into a range of antibiotic dilutions and incubated for 18 h. Cloudy tubes show inadequate inhibition of the organism (i.e. growth), while the clear ones indicate concentrations that prevent growth. The minimum inhibitory concentration is defined as the maximum dilution that prevents visible growth. Subsequent subculture of the clear tubes and comparison with the amount of growth in a tube containing broth without antibiotic allows determination of the concentration necessary to kill (rather than merely suppress) the inoculum. This defines the minimum bactericidal concentration

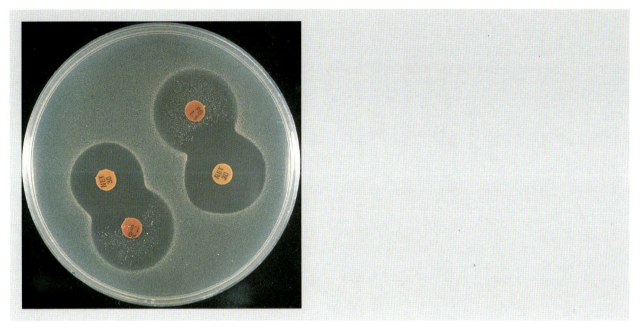

Figure 63 Demonstration of bactericidal synergy between benzylpenicillin (PG 1.5) and netilmicin (NET 30) by a layer-plate technique. The organism was inoculated onto the plate and the antibiotic discs added. After 18 h incubation, clear zones of inhibition round both discs are seen. The penicillin that has diffused into the surrounding medium is then destroyed by adding penicillinase, and the plates reincubated. The figure shows the regrowth of the organism in areas where penicillin alone had been acting. The absence of growth in the areas into which both anti-biotics had diffused demonstrates the bactericidal effect of the combination

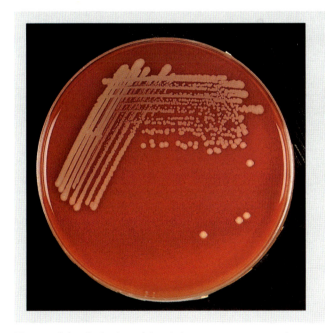

Figure 64 Colonies of *Staphylococcus aureus* growing on blood agar

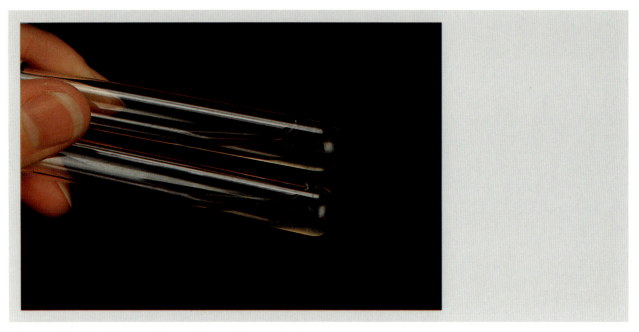

Figure 65 Identification of coagulase-positive staphylo-cocci. The ability to coagulate serum (lower tube) is characteristic of *Staphylococcus aureus*

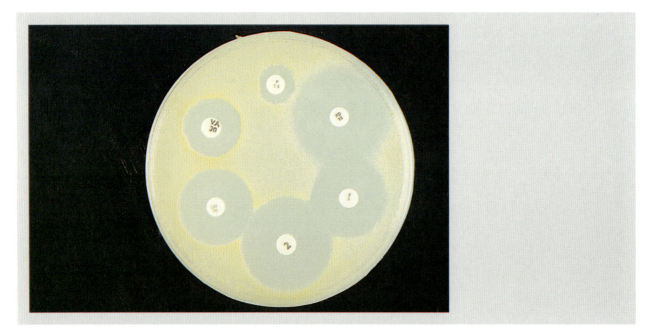

Figure 66 Penicillin (P)-resistant *Staphylococcus aureus* showing susceptibility to fucidin (FD), erythromycin (E), rifampicin (2), gentamicin (CN) and vancomycin (VA)

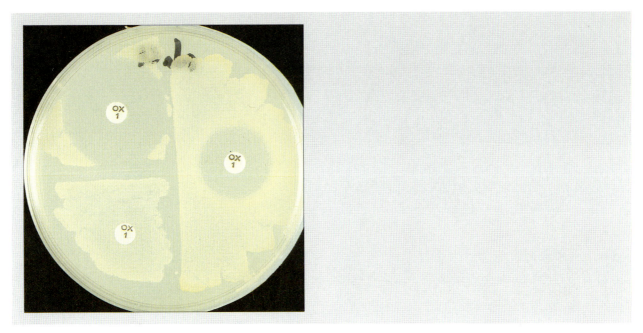

Figure 67 Determination of flucloxacillin susceptibility. Coagulase-positive staphylococci exhibit cross-sensitivity to isoxazolyl penicillin and methicillin. For technical reasons susceptibility testing has been carried out using oxacillin as the representative antibiotic of this group. The culture on the half-plate is the test isolate while the upper and lower quadrants contain standard susceptible and resistant isolates. Susceptibility to the antibiotic is indicated by inhibition of growth round the antibiotic-containing discs, and resistance by growth up to the disc

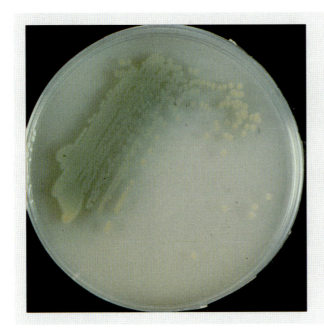

Figure 68 *Pseudomonas aeruginosa* growing on nutrient agar and showing development of green pigment by the bacterial colonies

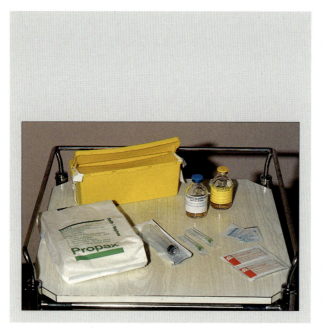

Figure 69 Assembly of the equipment required for collection of blood for culture, i.e. skin disinfectant, syringes, needles, culture bottles and sterile pack containing dressing towel, forceps etc.

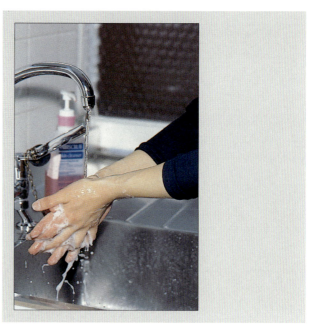

Figure 70 Thorough washing of the hands

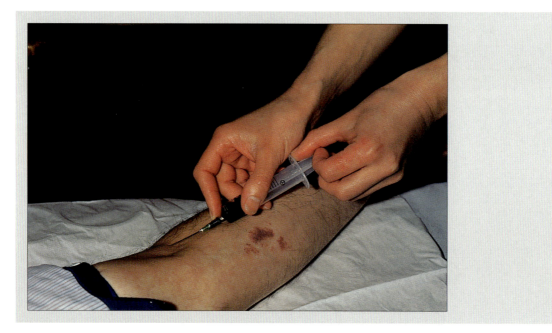

Figure 71 Venepuncture using the no-touch technique after the venepuncture site has been disinfected

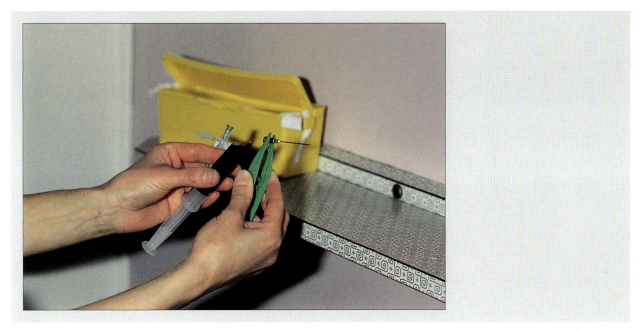

Figure 72   Needle change prior to inoculation of culture bottles

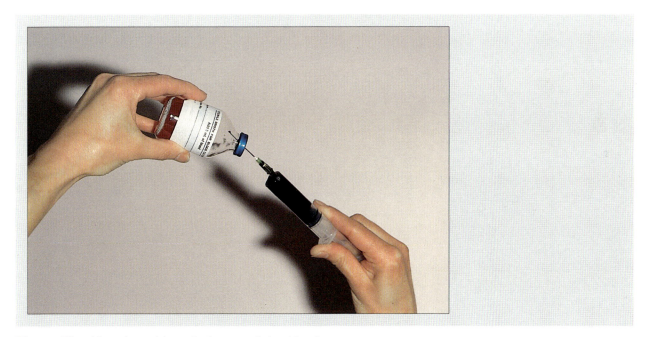

Figure 73   After the rubber diaphragm of the blood culture bottles has been disinfected (using an alcohol-based disinfectant) and allowed to dry, the recommended volume of blood is added to aerobic and anaerobic culture bottles

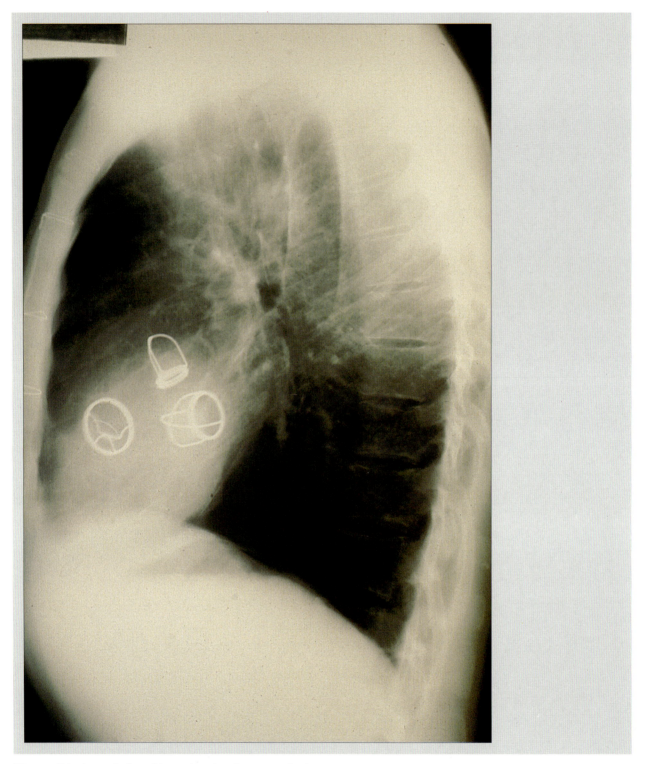

Figure 74 Lateral chest X-ray showing three prosthetic heart valves (tricuspid, aortic and mitral). A patient with a prosthetic heart valve has a 2%–4% chance of developing prosthetic valve endocarditis. The mortality is approximately 50%

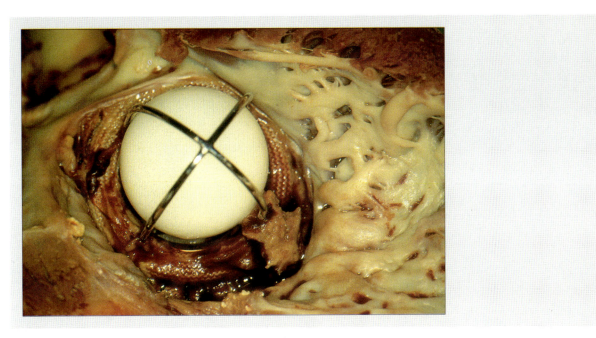

Figure 75 Starr Edwards aortic valve prosthesis. Infective endocarditis. Vegetations are clearly seen on the sewing ring of the valve

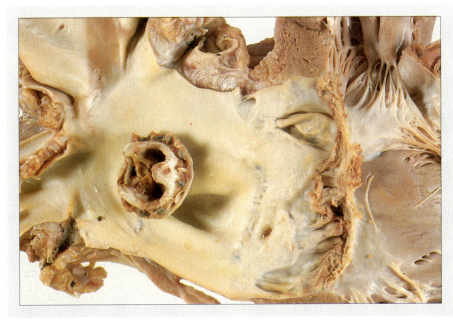

Figure 76 Prosthetic valve endocarditis. A 30-year-old patient appeared to be progressing well in response to antibiotics. After 2 weeks' treatment, echocardiography showed the development of valve rocking. She died sud- denly before surgery could be undertaken. At postmortem, the valve was seen to be completely detached from the aortic valve ring

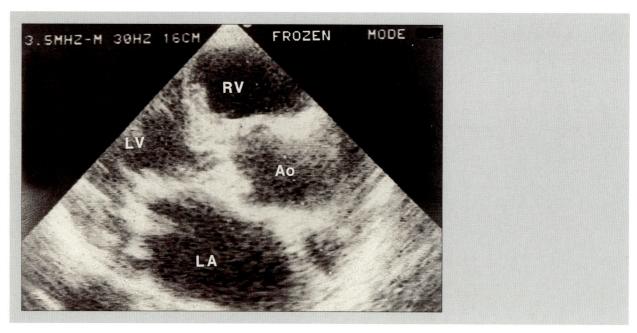

Figure 77 Transthoracic echocardiography – left parasternal long-axis view. The mitral valve is irregularly thickened with a mass protruding into the left atrium. The aortic valve is thickened

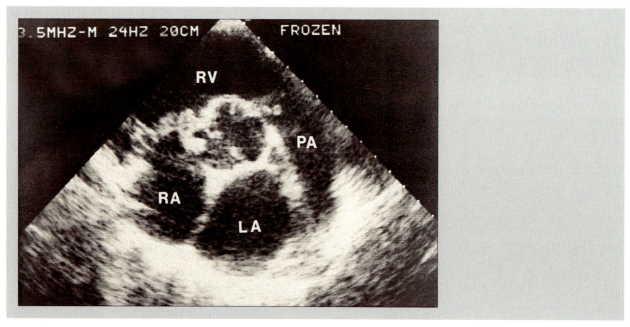

Figure 78 Right parasternal short-axis view of the same patient shown in Figure 77. Vegetations are present on the pulmonary, tricuspid and aortic valves

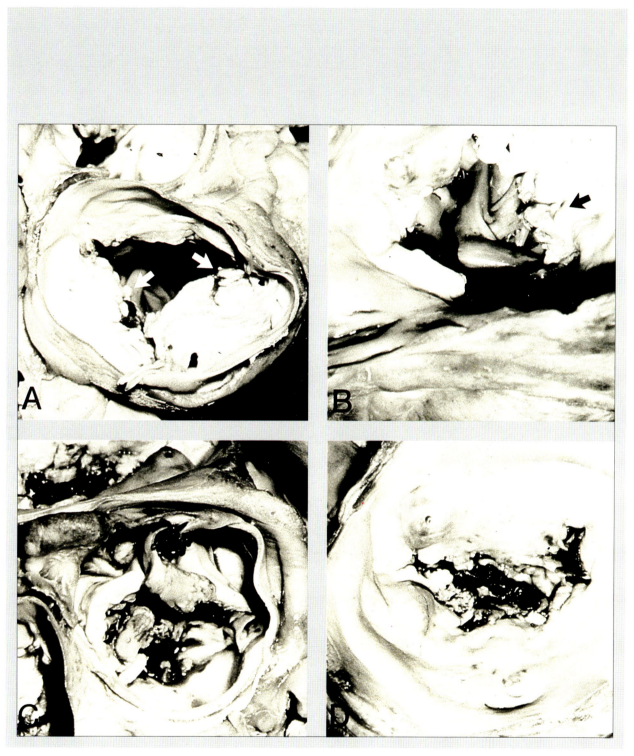

Figure 79 Same patient as shown in Figures 77 and 78. Valves as seen at postmortem examination. A. Pulmonary valve from above – vegetations on ventricular aspect. B. Tricuspid valve viewed from right atrium – a large vegetation is seen. C. Aortic valve viewed from above – multiple vegetations. D. Mitral valve viewed from left atrium – multiple vegetations. Spread of infection from one valve to another is quite common and of great practical importance in the context of surgical treatment. However, this case with infection of all four valves is unique

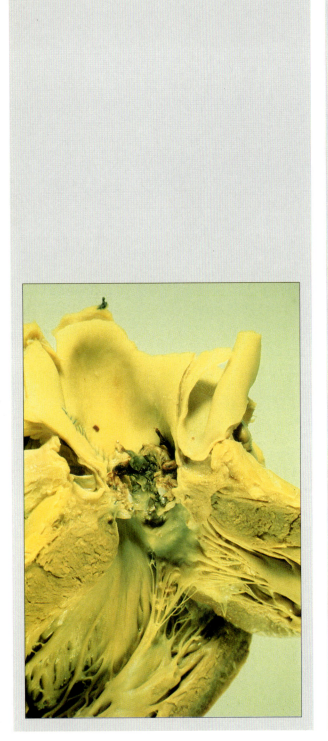

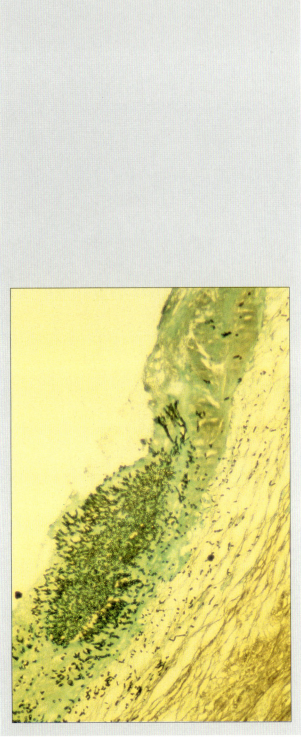

Figure 80 Fungal infection of a prosthetic tissue valve (*Aspergillus* spp.). Fungal endocarditis is uncommon and most cases are caused by *Candida* spp. This patient became ill 6 weeks after aortic valve replacement. A diagnosis of culture-negative endocarditis was made. He died 2 weeks later following a cerebral embolus

Figure 81 Microscopy of valve tissue from the patient shown in Figure 80 (methanamine silver stain). The fungi are stained black

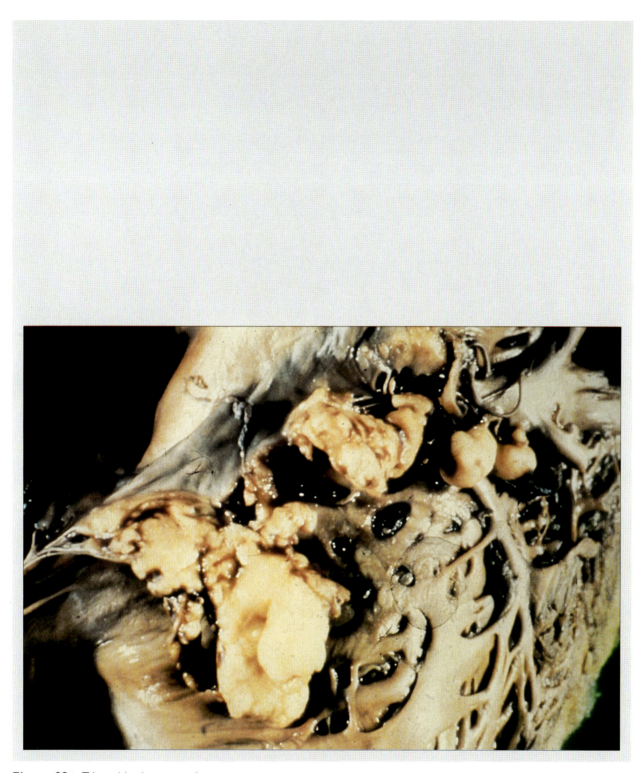

Figure 82   Tricuspid valve vegetations

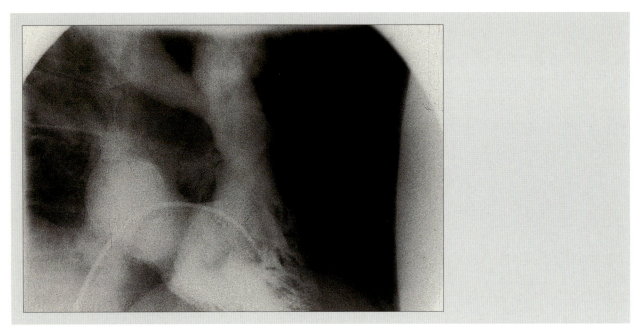

Figure 83 Right ventriculogram. Severe tricuspid regurgitation due to tricuspid endocarditis

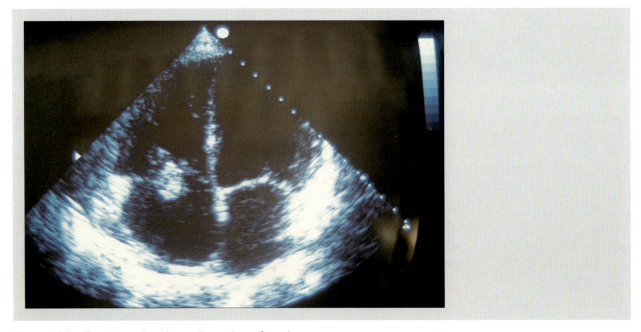

Figure 84 Transthoracic echocardiography – four-chamber view. Large vegetation clearly seen on the tricuspid valve. The patient, an elderly man, was not in a high-risk category. He was allergic to penicillin but responded well to a 4-week course of vancomycin

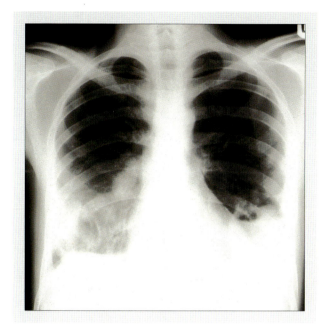

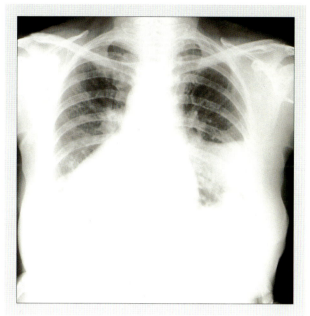

Figure 85 Chest X-ray showing lung abscesses. Air fluid levels can be seen. This was a 24-year-old male heroin addict with a history of chills and a productive cough. Tricuspid valve endocarditis caused by *Staphylococcus aureus* was treated with flucloxacillin and netilmicin. Four years later his exercise tolerance was normal. The prognosis in this group of patients is generally good

Figure 86 Chest X-ray. Radiological findings consistent with pulmonary embolism. In this case, right basal atelectasis is shown. Similar changes can be seen on an initial chest X-ray in approximately 50% of patients with tricuspid valve endocarditis

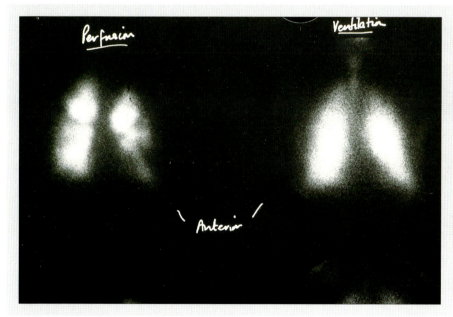

Figure 87 V/Q scan. There is marked ventilation perfusion mismatch shown by several defects in the perfusion scan not seen in the ventilation scan. This is indicative of multiple pulmonary emboli

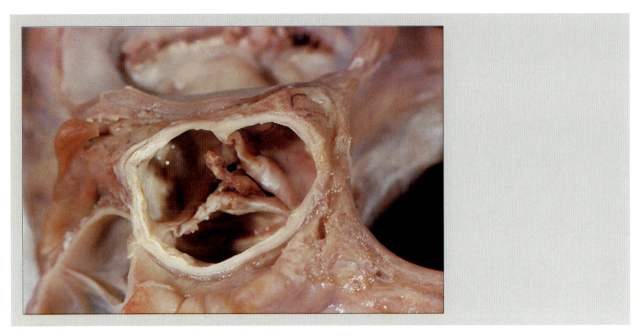

Figure 88 Aortic valve endocarditis caused by *Chlamydia psittaci* (psittacosis). A large finger-like vegetation is projecting through the aortic valve into the root of the aorta. This is one cause of culture-negative endocarditis

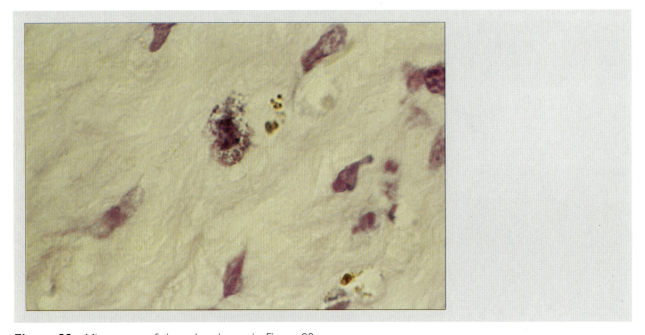

Figure 89 Microscopy of the valve shown in Figure 88 (× 400) using Machieavello stain. Characteristic intracellular inclusions are shown (Leventhal–Cole–Lille bodies)

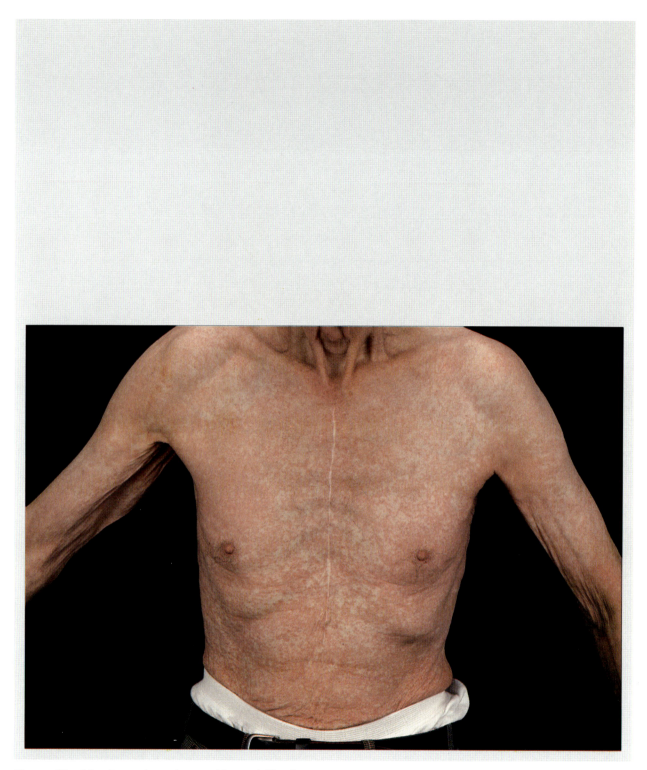

Figure 90   Maculopapular rash caused by penicillin allergy in a patient with prosthetic valve endocarditis (note median sternotomy scar). Penicillin allergy is often accompanied by a low-grade pyrexia and sometimes also by neutropenia

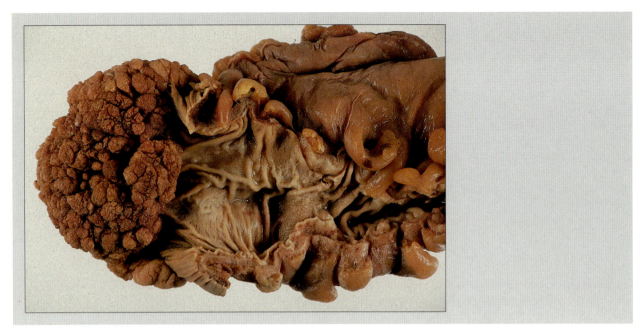

Figure 91   Benign villous adenoma (polyp) of colon

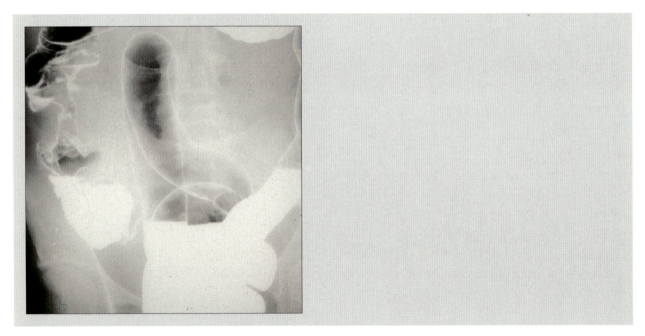

Figure 92   Barium enema showing filling defects due to carcinoma of the ascending colon. A malignant or premalignant bowel lesion is present in up to 75% of patients who have endocarditis caused by *Streptococcus bovis*. Barium enema and/or colonoscopy is indicated in all patients with endocarditis caused by this organism

Section 3   Bibliography

Anderson, D. G. and Reefer, C. S. (1948). *The Therapeutic Value of Penicillin*. (Ann Arbor Michegan: J. W. Edwards)

Bayer, A. S. and Theofilopoulos, A. N. (1990). Immunopathological aspects of infective endocarditis. *Chest*, **97**, 204–12

Boyd, A. D., Spencer, F. C., Isom, O. W., Cunningham, J. N., Reed, G. E., Acinapura, A. J. and Tice, D. A. (1977). Infective endocarditis: an analysis of 54 surgically treated patients. *J. Thorac. Cardiovasc. Surg.*, **73**, 23–9

Braunwald, E. (1992). Heart Disease. *A Textbook of Cardiovascular Medicine*, 4th edn. (Philadelphia, London, Toronto, Montreal, Sydney, Tokyo: W. B. Saunders Company)

Byrd, B. F., Shelton, M. E., Wilson, B. H. and Schillig, S. (1990). Infective perivalvular abscess of the aortic ring: echocardiographic features and clinical course. *Am. J. Cardiol.*, **66**, 102–5

Calderwood, S. B., Swinski, L. A., Waternaux, C. M., Kratchmer, A. W. and Buckley, M. J. (1985). Risk factors for the development of prosthetic valve endocarditis. *Circulation*, **72**, 31–7

Cardullo, A. C., Silvers, D. N. and Grossman, M. E. (1990). Janeway lesions & Osler's nodes: a review of histopathological findings. *J. Am. Acad. Dermatol.*, **22**, 1088–90

Counsell, C. E., de Belder, M. A. and Oldershaw, P. J. (1991). Prosthetic valve endocarditis. *Br. J. Hosp. Med.*, **46**, 28–31

Dismukes, W. E., Kratchmer, A. W., Buckley, M. J., Austen, W. G. and Schwartz, M. N. (1973). Prosthetic valve endocarditis: analysis of 38 cases. *Circulation*, **48**, 365–77

Douglas, A., Moore-Gillon, J. and Eykyn, S. (1986). Fever during treatment of infective endocarditis. *Lancet*, **1**, 1341–3

Dupuis, G., Peter, O., Luthy, R., Nicolet, J., Peacock, M. and Burgdorfer, W. (1986). Serological diagnosis of Q fever endocarditis. *Eur. Heart J.*, **7**, 1062–6

Espersen, F. and Frimodt-Moller, N. (1986). *Staphylococcus aureus* endocarditis. A review of 119 cases. *Arch. Int. Med.*, **146**, 1118–21

Gleckler, W. J. (1960). Subacute bacterial endocarditis in old person. *Geriatrics*, **15**, 152–7

Goodwin, J. F. (1985). The challenge vs. the reproach of infective endocarditis. (Editorial). *Br. Heart J.*, **54**, 115–18

Gossius, G., Gunnes, P. and Rasmussen, K. (1985). Ten years of infective endocarditis. A clinicopathological study. *Acta Med. Scand.*, **217**, 171–9

Gray, I. R. (1991). Rational approach to the treatment of culture negative infective endocarditis. *Drugs*, **41**, 729–36

Hampton, J. R. and Harrison, M. J. G. (1967). Sterile blood cultures in bacterial endocarditis. *Quart. J. Med.*, **36**, 167–74

Hecht, S. R. and Berger, M. (1992). Right-sided endocarditis in intravenous drug users. *Ann. Int. Med.*, **117**, 560–6

Horstkotte, D. and Bodnar, E. (1991). *Current Issues in Heart Valve Disease: Infective Endocarditis*. (London: ICR Publishers)

Hughes, P. and Gauld, W. R. C. (1966). Bacterial endocarditis: a changing disease. *Quart. J. Med.*, **35**, 511–20

Jones, H. R. and Siekert, R. G. (1989). Neurological manifestations of infective endocarditis. *Brain*, **112**, 1295–315

Kaye, D. (1973). Changes in the spectrum diagnosis and management of bacterial and fungal endocarditis. *Med. Clin. N. Am.*, **57**, 941–56

Kaye, D. (1985). Changing pattern of infective endocarditis. *Am. J. Med.*, **78**, (Suppl. 6B), 157–61

Khan, S. S. and Gray, R. J. (1991). Valvular emergencies. *Cardiology Clin.*, **9**, (No. 4), 689–94

Kratchmer, A. W. (1991). Prosthetic valve endocarditis: a continuing challenge for infection control. *J. Hosp. Inf.*, **18**, (Suppl. A.), 355–66

Editorial. (1984). Infective endocarditis. *Lancet*, **1**, 603–4

Lerner, P. I. and Weinstein, L. (1966). Medical progress. Infective endocarditis in the antibiotic era. *N. Engl. J. Med.*, **274**, 199–206

Major, R. H. (1978). *Classic Descriptions of Disease*, 3rd edn. (Illinois: Thomas Springfield)

Manhas, D. R., Mohri, H., Hessel, G. A. and Merendind, K. A. (1972). Experience with surgical management of primary infective endocarditis: a collected review of 139 patients. *Am. Heart J.*, **84**, 738–47

Mayer, E.-D., Ruffman, K., Saggau, W., Butzmann, B., Bernhardt-Mayer, K., Schatton, N. and Schmitz, W. (1985). Ruptured aneurysms of the Sinus of Valsalva. *Ann. Thorac. Surg.*, **42**, 81–5

Megran, D. W. (1992). Enterococcal endocarditis. *Clin. Inf. Dis.*, **15**, 63–71

Morganroth, J., Perloff, J. K., Zeldis, S. M. and Dunkman, W. B. (1977). Acute severe aortic regurgitation. *Ann. Int. Med.*, **87**, 223–32

Nanda, N. C. (1989). *Atlas of Colour Doppler Echocardiography*. (Philadelphia and London: Lea and Febiger)

Osler, W. (1885). Malignant endocarditis. *Lancet*, **1**, 459–64

Popp, R. L. (1990). Echocardiography. *N. Engl. J. Med.*, **323**, 165–72

Rutledge, R., Kim, B. J. and Applebaum, R. E. (1985). Actuarial analysis of the risk of prosthetic valve endocarditis in 1598 patients with mechanical and bioprosthetic valves. *Arch. Surg.*, **120**, 469–72

Schnurr, L. P., Ball, A. P., Geddes, A. M., Gray, J. and McGhie, D. (1977). Bacterial endocarditis in England in the 1970s. A review of 70 patients. *Quart. J. Med.*, **46**, 499–512

Seldin, E. B. (1985). Dental factors in infective endocarditis. (Editorial). *Circulation*, **71**, 1093–4

Slaughter, L., Morris, J. E. and Starr, A. (1973). Prosthetic valvular endocarditis. A 12 year review. *Circulation*, **47**, 1319–26

Stinson, E. B., Griepp, R. B., Vosti, K., Copeland, J. G. and Shumway, N. E. (1976). Operative treatment of active endocarditis. *J. Thorac. Cardiovasc. Surg.*, **71**, 659–64

Taams, M. A., Gussenhoven, E. J., Bos, E., de Jaegere, P., Roelandt, J. R. T. C., Sutherland, G. R. and Bom, N. (1990). Enhanced morphological diagnosis in infective endocarditis by transoesophageal echocardiography. *Br. Heart J.*, **63**, 109–13

Ward, C., Jephcott, A. E. and Hardisty, C. A. (1977). Perioperative antibiotic prophylaxis and prosthetic valve endocarditis. *Postgrad. Med. J.*, **53**, 1–3

Whitby, M. and Fenech, A. (1985). Infective endocarditis in adults in Glasgow 1976–87. *Int. J. Cardiol.*, **7**, 391–403

White, P. D. (1945). *Heart Disease*, 3rd edn. (New York: The Macmillan Company)

Index

abscess
  Brodie's 46
  cerebral 23, 24, 33, 52
  detection of 27, 28, 70
  lung 85
  myocardial 22–23
  paravulvar 23, 27, 28, 70
allergy 34, 87
angiography 28, 68, 69
antimicrobial
  susceptibility testing 73, 74
  therapy 15, 33–34
aortic valve 43
  endocarditis 48–49, 51, 80–81, 86
  incidence 16
  regurgitation 17, 68–70
aortogram 68–69
aneurysm 23, 24, 34
  aortic 34
  detection of 27, 28
  mycotic 23, 24

bacteria 26, see also organism
bacteremia 19–21, 28
barium enema 88
blood cultures 25, 76–77

cardiac failure
  management 33
  significance 22
cardiac involvement 21–23

chest X-rays 28
  adult respiratory distress syndrome 51
  lung abscesses 85
  prosthetic heart valves 78
  pulmonary edema 51
  pulmonary embolism 85
chordae tendineae rupture 22, 50, 65
clinical features
  anemia 28
  bacteremia 19–20
  cardiac 21–23, 30
  cutaneous 24, 56, 57
  general 20, 28, 31
  subconjunctival hemorrhage 24, 56
complications
  abscesses, see abscess
  adult respiratory distress syndrome 51
  aneurysm 23, 24, 27, 28, 34
  cardiac failure 22, 33, 50, 51
  central nervous system involvement 23–24, 52
  embolic, see emboli
  renal 24, 28, 54–55
  endocardiographic detection 23, 27
computer tomography (CT) 28, 33, 52
coronary heart disease 28
culture-negative endocarditis 26, 32, 58
cutaneous manifestations 24, 56, 57

degenerative valve disease 21–22, 45
dental caries 19, 47

diagnosis 19–20
  blood cultures 25–26
  differential diagnosis 24, 30, 58, 59
  atrial myxoma 24, 59
  systemic lupus erythematosus 24, 58
  thrombotic thrombocytopenic purpura 24
drug addicts 16, 19, 31

echocardiography 23, 27–28, 33–34, 59, 67, 80, 81
  M mode 27, 59, 67
  transesophageal 27, 30, 60–62, 64–66, 70
  with prosthetic valve endocarditis 27, 30, 66, 70
elderly patients 31–32
emboli 20, 21, 23, 33
  cerebral 23, 82
  coronary 22
  pulmonary 85
  renal 24, 54, 55
  splenic 53
  with fungal endocarditis 31
  with prosthetic valve endocarditis 29
endocarditis
  culture negative 32, 86
  etiology 17, 22
  iatrogenic 19, 29, 47
  intravenous drug abuse 19, 31
  management 33–34
  native valve, see under valve, name
  prosthetic valve 29–30, 78, 79
epidemiology 16, 19, 31

fever, during treatment 34
fungal endocarditis 26, 30, 32, 82

glomerulonephritis 24, 28, 54, 55

historical notes 15–16

immunocompromised patients 16, 19, 30
  fungal endocarditis and 30
immunological responses 28
investigation 25–28
  abdominal ultrasound 28, 53
  angiography 28

C-reactive protein measurement 28
chest X-rays 28, 33, 51, 78, 85
computerized tomography 28
echocardiography 27–28
leukocytosis 28, 29
microbiological 25–26
urinalysis 28

management 33–34
microbiology 25–26
mortality rates 15, 16
  late deaths 34
murmur 22, 30, 34, 50
myxoma, atrial 24, 67, 59

non-bacterial thrombotic endocarditis 17, 24, 41–43

organisms 26
  aspergillus 30, 82
  brucella 26, 32
  candida 26, 30, 82
  chlamydia 26, 32, 86
  coxiella 26, 32
  diptheroids 26
  enterococcus 26
  gram negative 16
  haemophilus 21
  legionella 26, 32
  Q fever 26, 32
  staphylococcus 16, 21, 23, 26, 48, 49, 85
  streptococcus 17, 21, 26, 72, 88
Osler nodes 20, 57
osteomyelitis 19, 46

pacemaker infection 47
pathogenesis
  adhesion of bacteria 17
  non-bacterial thrombotic 24, 41–43
  predisposing lesions
    bicuspid aortic valve 22, 45, 49
    congenital heart lesions 21–22
    degenerative valve disease 22, 31
    mitral valve prolapse 44
    patent ductus 17, 22

rheumatic heart disease 21–22
bacteremia 19–21, 28, 31
  colonic adenoma 88
  dental 19, 47
  drug abuse 16, 19, 31
prosthetic 29–30, 78, 79

rash 24, 34, 56, 57, 87
renal involvement 24, 28, 54–55
  renal failure, chronic 31
  renal infarction 54
rheumatic fever 24
rheumatic heart disease 21–22
rheumatic endocarditis 15, 58
Roth spot 24, 57

skin manifestations 24, *see also* rash
surgery
  indications for 16, 22, 33, 34

mortality 16
symptoms 21–24

valve
  aortic 22, 43
  mitral 43
    chordae tendineae rupture 22, 50, 65
    prolapse 21–22, 44
    regurgitation 17, 22, 65
    intracardiac pressure tracings 50
    left ventriculogram 68
    vegetations 48, 80–81
  prosthetic 29–30, 79
  pulmonary 80–81
  replacement of 16, 22, 33, 34
  tricuspid 33, 80, 81, 83, 85
vegetations 15, 17, 27, 41

X-rays 28, 33, 51, 78, 85